The
Holistic
Health
Movement

The
Holistic
Health
Movement

Kristine Beyerman Alster

The University of Alabama Press

Tuscaloosa and London

Library of Congress Cataloging-in-Publication Data

Alster, Kristine Beyerman.
  The holistic health movement.

  Bibliography: p.
  Includes index.
  1. Holistic medicine—Philosophy.   2. Holistic
medicine—History.   I. Title. [DNLM: 1. Holistic
Health. W 61 A463h]
R733.A45 1989   613   88–14278
ISBN 0–8173–0416–9 (alk. paper)

British Library Cataloging-in-Publication Data is available.

For Norm

My Sweetheart
and Husband

Contents

Acknowledgments

It is very gratifying to have an opportunity to thank publicly some of the people who helped me as I worked on this book. Victor Kestenbaum, of Boston University, encouraged me to believe that the ideas in a short paper on the holistic health movement had merit and could be expanded into a larger work. As a dissertation adviser, he made demands that felt like invitations—to learn, to challenge fixed ideas, to see the larger implications of a practice or a belief. The other two members of my dissertation committee also contributed a great deal to the development of this volume. Margery Chisholm, a nurse and psychotherapist, offered significant insights into the impact of the holistic health movement on the health professions. Bruce McPherson spent hours discussing the social implications of the movement with me; it was he who first suggested that the health beliefs of holists could be characterized as slogans.

A number of individuals associated with The University of Alabama Press were generous with their help: Director Malcolm MacDonald guided me through the review process; two anonymous reviewers suggested some important changes in the manuscript; and Robert G. Ferris gracefully edited the final text.

Finally, let me say yet another thanks in a series of thanks that goes back years—to my family and friends, who were lovingly patient even when it seemed that there would *never* be a final draft.

The
Holistic
Health
Movement

Introduction

At one time, "health" as a noun seldom required any adjective other than "good" or "bad." Now it seems there is a new kind of health: holistic health. The term indicates that the health being qualified is better some how than merely good health.

It is being celebrated everywhere: on television and in print, in schools, churches, and clinics. It has supporters among fringe groups, cultists, and mystics as well as among the lay public and health professionals. Organizations such as the American Holistic Medical Association, American Holistic Nurses Association, and Holistic Dental Association International have been established. As one source says, "The words *holism* and *holistic* are being tossed about as enthusiastically as a frisbee in the springtime" (Albright, P. and B. P., 1980, p. ix).

In the growing holistic literature, a sense of discovery and excitement is accompanied by an almost evangelical desire to spread the word. Advocates are eager to share their perspective, which they believe provides a superior understanding of man and his health. At times, this enthusiasm becomes rather strident. Some believe that the holistic approach is not simply interesting, but correct.

1

It is they who have introduced an unfortunate tone of smugness to the literature.

The "cheerleaders" draw our attention; the self-righteous disciples make us wary. But the holistic health movement cannot be ignored. The promises it makes are too intriguing. Any movement that claims it can restructure the way we think about health and illness (Fink, 1980), revolutionize the health-care delivery system (Carlson, 1981), and vastly improve our health (Travis, 1980a) is a force to be reckoned with. Although it may or may not be true that the "shift toward holism is really irreversible" (Carlson, 1981, p. 509), it is certainly influencing our attitudes, behavior, and expectations at the present. Given the current level of interest, it is reasonable to assume that such influence will continue to be felt for some time.

Even those who do not march under the banner of the "movement" find themselves affected by it. Much of the current interest in fitness and exercise can be traced to it, as can the concern about food additives and a healthy diet. The notion of medical self-help was the offspring of the consumer and holistic health movements. Even the conventional Blue Cross-Blue Shield group reflects the trend in its "Health Thyself" ads.

Is the holistic health movement merely a fad that has momentarily tickled the national fancy? Certainly it has some of the earmarks of a fad in view of its sudden popularity and voguish vocabulary. But it would be a mistake to dismiss it too lightly because it deals with the important issues of health and illness. Although the term "holistic health" is relatively new, the problems it seeks to address are old indeed, for mankind has long sought the means to secure good health. Nor are the cardinal tenets of the movement new; modern holistic health advocates are not the first to suggest that man is a complex, inte-

grated organism whose health is affected by myriad influences, many of which are under his own control.

Although some of its manifestations are patently silly,
the phenomenon must be regarded as something more
than a fad. Even if the term "holistic health" does not
survive the decade, it will leave a residue of beliefs, values, and practices that will continue to affect our ideas
about health and health care well into the future.

Any phenomenon that touches our lives in this way
deserves a respectful hearing; it requires a careful and
critical analysis as well. The holistic health movement
has had the former. It has been acknowledged by the lay
public, by various professional groups, and by such government agencies as the National Institute of Mental
Health (Hastings, Fadiman, and Gordon, 1981). But, although there has been much in the way of celebration,
there has been little thoughtful analysis.

Indeed, it is tempting to subscribe to a system that has
such lofty goals and promises such sunny benefits: better
health, improved care at lower cost, a more egalitarian
relationship between client and provider, control over
our own welfare, peace of mind. These promises have
caught our imagination. Arthur O. Lovejoy has said:

> You may . . . find much of the thinking of an individual,
> a school, or even a generation, dominated and deter-
> mined by one or another turn of reasoning, trick of logic,
> methodological assumption, which if explicit would
> amount to a large and important and perhaps highly de-
> batable proposition in logic or metaphysics. (in Phillips,
> 1976, unnumbered page facing p.1)

Phillips has used this quote to suggest that holistic
thought is such a "turn of reasoning."

The appeal of the holistic health movement is obvious

and it is strong. In spite of that appeal, or rather because of it, we need to examine it closely, lest we be seduced by a system that promises more than it can deliver.

Holistic health has, of course, had its critics, mostly among physicians. One cannot help wondering if this is because that group stands to lose the most by a change in the status quo of health care. The feeling of threat was evident in the hyperbole used by one physician who likened the proliferation of holistic practices to "an uncontrolled nuclear reaction" (Callan, 1979, p. 1156). But legitimate issues have been raised. Lange (1980) has suggested that unorthodox practices and unlicensed clinicians make the public vulnerable to charlatans and quackery. Block (1981) warns that, in their eagerness to identify the mental and emotional components of illness, some holists may overlook significant physical problems. A serious concern among many doctors is that practitioners who embrace a holistic philosophy will turn away from the most helpful contributions of conventional medicine (Frank, 1981).

Other health-care professionals have voiced doubts. Greene (1981) has asked whether it is appropriate for dentists to treat "the whole person," as some of his colleagues have suggested. Chinn, a nurse, suggests that the concept of holism needs further development: "Much of the literature focusing on holistic health appears superficial, vague, inexact, subjective and generally inconsistent with traditional values upon which science is based" (1980, p. xii).

But the individual voices of caution and dissent have been overwhelmed by the chorus of approval heard in the health-care literature. Many writers do not even attempt to justify the use of a holistic framework. It may be taken for granted that holism is a good, even the only, frame of reference. In some circles, it is almost necessary to baptize one's work as holistic before presenting it to the reader. No further reference to holism may be made, but the initial acknowledgment is obligatory.

To fail to make it is to render one's writing vulnerable to attack. A case in point is the review conducted by two registered nurses of articles written by psychiatric nurses (Oleck and Yoder, 1981). Entitled "Holism or Hypocrisy," it was critical of those articles that the researchers felt did not adequately reflect a holistic approach to the practice of psychiatric nursing.

This book offers a critical analysis of the movement. I will attempt to articulate the ideas and values that are central to holistic health, and will evaluate their usefulness and significance for health care. I am particularly interested in what might be termed "mainstream holistic health." Although the movement was partly an outgrowth of the counterculture, it has steadily gained acceptance by conventional health-care practitioners and recognition by the scientific as well as academic communities. This volume will focus on holistic health as defined and practiced by these groups. The efficacy of various therapies and techniques espoused by holistic practitioners will not be discussed except incidentally. This study will not be concerned with the tools of holistic health, but rather with its philosophy.

First, the history of the movement will be outlined, and some of the major contributions to its thinking from the natural sciences, philosophy, psychology, the human potential movement, and the counterculture will be identified. Although the movement remains rather amorphous and ill-defined, an attempt will be made to outline the major elements of its thinking. The shared values, beliefs, and assumptions of holists exert an influence beyond the boundaries of the movement itself, and for this reason it should be carefully scrutinized. Few of us remain unexposed to holistic thought, even if we do not identify it as such. Herein lies the potential peril of accepting as received wisdom that which may be flawed, even dangerous or unhealthy. Some of what comes to us from the movement has value; some does not. The following chapters will examine the impact of holistic thought on our understanding of the nature of health, on the individual and his efforts to maintain health, on our society and the values it associates with health, and on the health-care professions.

1

The Origins of Modern Holistic Thought

It has been said that it is always perilous to attempt to assign an exact origin for any scientific idea, because when we think that we have traced its history back to a dark age that must surely have marked its inception, we shall still probably find that if we go back but a little further, and again a little further, the previously assigned origin does not seem to be so definite after all. The idea does not appear to have sprung, Athena-like out of a placid background, as we may have first thought. Its roots lie buried in a soil that is very, very deep.

(Commins, 1932, p. 208)

The relationship between mind and body has intrigued mankind throughout the ages. From the pre-Socratics to present scholars, thinkers in many fields have considered the nature of man and offered theories and models to explain his complexity. Man's experienced sense of himself as something other, something *more*, than a machine or a lump of tissue has led him into endless speculation regarding the nature of the connection between his body and the "other."

Philosophers have long quarreled about the essential nature of man and his relationship to the universe. Psychologists have investigated the relationship of his body to subjective internal states, physicians have observed the association of physical function and behavior, and theologians have promulgated dogma regarding body and soul.

Assumptions about the mind-body connection have changed over time, during which various degrees of dualism or holism have reigned as the dominant mode. Even in those periods when dualism was in the ascendancy, however, holistic thought was still to be found in the writings of the time.

Modern proponents of holistic health care seem only faintly aware of the currents of historical thought on which their movement is based. In some popular works on the subject, holism is celebrated as something novel, unique to our times, an invention of the late twentieth century. Many authors have described its thinking as representing a new "paradigm" in health care (Capra, 1982; Ferguson, M., 1980; Flynn, 1980). Borrowing from Kuhn's (1970) work, they suggest that a holistic approach to health care is so original that it qualifies as a paradigm shift, that is, an entirely new way of characterizing and approaching the problems of a given discipline.

Although some of the practices used may be new (and not all are), the notion of man as an integrated being is not, nor is the belief that his health can be improved by a practitioner who acknowledges his essential wholeness. Many voices have supported these ideas; many healers have used them. Thus, it is a misuse of Kuhn's concept to nominate the current appearance of holism as a paradigm shift in health care.

Even those who understand that holism is not a product of the 1980s sometimes demonstrate considerable confusion about its origins. Gordon (1981) actually claimed that "the concept of 'holism' was first introduced by the South African philosopher Jan Christian Smuts in 1926" (p. 3). Although Smuts coined the term, he certainly did not introduce the concept, the roots of which indeed go very deep. Holists display a remarkable naiveté when they fail to recognize themselves as part of a long and complex tradition.

Furthermore, those who do avoid the ahistorical perspective of their colleagues give short shrift to the complexity of the issues as well as the important and insistent claims of the opposition. Zaner (1981) notes that "dualism . . . is not merely one of the passing points of view which pop in and out of the historical panorama of metaphysics, like some wacky Punch and Judy show. Nor is it simply an intractably persistent *bête noir*, forever dogging the tracks of monism's thrust to more pristine regions, where one might hope to be ethereally innocent of the vexing questions of otherness" (pp. 6–7). Yet, this is the dominant attitude among today's holists. They have forsaken the tradition of struggle, debate, and honest engagement of the issue.

This chapter will examine that tradition and discuss some of the contributions made by various disciplines. My intent is to demonstrate that the ideas subscribed to by modern holists have not "sprung Athena-like out of a placid background." In no way will I attempt to construct a comprehensive history of holism—that task is too large for the purposes of this book. Rather, some of the major sources from which the modern holistic health movement has drawn inspiration will be analyzed.

Even this more modest task appears formidable when one considers the span of time and the number of disciplines involved. Furthermore, holistic thinkers appear to have delighted in creating idiosyncratic vocabularies so that the modern reader must struggle to identify parallels. What, for example, is the relationship between "the One" of Parmenides and Spinoza's "Nature"? And how does Hegel's "Essential Relation" correspond to the Yin and Yang of Chinese thought?

D. C. Phillips has pointed out some of the difficulties encountered by the student of holism:

> There is an enormous body of literature on holism, but a student . . . is unlikely to encounter it in any ordered way. He is almost certain to meet at least a few holistic theses, and probably some of the arguments against them; but he is likely to remain ignorant of the full scope of holism. He may not realize that the debates over methodological individualism or the place of psychological explanations in sociology are related to those over system theory, over organicism in biology and psychology, over structuralism and functionalism, and over internal relations in philosophy. And he can easily become confused: the difficulty of finding a clear statement of the central ideas of holism in the literature is notorious, and there is a corresponding difficulty in evaluating them. (1976, pp. 1–2)

Given such a disorderly history, it is inevitable that my sketch of it will be somewhat untidy as well. It will be selective, using for the most part only major participants in the dialogue. It will be arbitrary in its classifications. Descartes, for example, will be discussed as a scientist and not as a philosopher; James as a philosopher and not a psychologist. And it will not be strictly linear in its progression because the development of holistic thought has been so convoluted. It will begin, in fact, in the middle—where the holists themselves usually begin—with that arch-villain of dualism, René Descartes.

Descartes, Medicine, and the Natural Sciences

Some holists have cleaved history into two parts: before and after Descartes. To them, the Age of Enlightenment in Europe initiated the holistic Dark Ages. They
paint a picture of a world in which an integrated model
of man was universally accepted and in which health care
and medicine were guided by holistic principles. Into this
holistic Eden came Descartes, bearing the apple of dualism. Discarding any notions of the harmony and unity
of the human organism, he substituted in their stead a
conception of the body and mind as separate and distinct, thereby wreaking havoc on a health-care system
previously distinguished by its orderly balance of psyche, soma, and their surroundings. One writer offers this
description:

> The greatest change in the history of Western medicine
> came with the Cartesian revolution. Before Descartes,
> most healers had addressed themselves to the interplay
> of body and soul, and had treated their patients within
> the context of their social and spiritual environment. As
> their world views changed over the ages, so did their
> views of illness and their methods of treatment, but their
> approaches were usually concerned with the whole pa-
> tient. Descartes' philosophy changed this situation pro-
> foundly. His strict division between mind and body led
> physicians to concentrate on the body machine and to
> neglect psychological, social, and environmental aspects
> of illness. (Capra, 1982, p. 126)

Descartes's far-reaching effect on medicine cannot be
denied. His influence on all the natural sciences has been
tremendous. It has been noted that, "though he was not
a physician in the strict sense of the word, [he had] an

unusually deep and lasting impact on the development of medicine" (Lindeboom, 1978, Preface). Nevertheless, it is ingenuous to suggest, as some holists do, that holistic thought in medicine was destroyed by Descartes and only resurrected four centuries later. Likewise, the proposition that all health care had a holistic orientation prior to the 1600s cannot be supported. (This idea of holistic medicine as an ancient but forgotten mode of practice stands in odd contradiction to the notion of a "new paradigm" mentioned earlier.) Although it must be acknowledged that Descartes's dualism occasioned a sharp shift toward a mechanistic biology and medicine, not all of his predecessors thought in holistic terms; neither did all of his followers subscribe to his dualism.

Indeed, it has been suggested by La Mettrie and others that Descartes himself believed in a unified model of man and deliberately misrepresented himself in his writings so as to avoid the wrath of the Church. Spicker (1970) claims that "it is simply one of the ironies of the history of European philosophy that Descartes is not a 'Cartesian' " (p. 9).

Nevertheless, that model which has come to be called Cartesian dualism, regardless of whether or not it accurately reflects Descartes's own beliefs, has occupied a remarkable place in Western thought. It had a profound impact on the evolution of the central themes of the Enlightenment. These themes—which include the superiority of rational over intuitive or mystical modes of thought, the primacy of the natural sciences, the search for a single system capable of explaining all phenomena from human behavior to the movement of the stars—continue to be significant themes today (Berlin, 1980). This is taken as evidence by certain holists of the hegemony of Cartesian dualism for the past four centuries.

But, as Berlin notes, "opposition to the central ideas of the French Enlightenment, and of its allies and disciples in other European countries, is as old as the movement itself" (p. 1). He points out that many voices were raised in protest and suggests that, rather than being an isolated occurrence, it was an instance of the backlash of mysticism and antirationalism that frequently followed the rise of rationalist thought (p. 82). A brief look at medical history demonstrates that in this field too, contrary to the popular holistic view, holistic and dualistic theories have always competed for dominance.

Hippocrates, recognized as the father of Western medicine, is sometimes cited as an example of an early holistic practitioner; and, indeed, many of his works support this claim. He believed that the brain was the seat of emotions as well as the cause of behavior and that it could be influenced by bodily events. Physical disorders, and not demons, were responsible for madness:

> Thus is this disease formed and prevails from those things which enter into and go out of the body. . . . And men ought to know that from nothing else but thence (*from the brain*) come joys, delights, laughter and sports, and sorrows, griefs, despondency, and lamentations. . . . As long as the brain is at rest, the man enjoys his reason, but the depravement of the brain arises from phlegm and bile. (Hippocrates, 1939, p. 366)

In addition to believing that the relationship between mind and body affected health, Hippocrates supposed that environmental factors were significant as well. In his book *On Airs, Waters, and Places*, he discusses how illness can arise from inappropriate conditions.

Nevertheless, the organicism of the Hippocratic writings did not go unchallenged. Brock states that, "impressed by this view of the organism as a unity, the Hippocratic school tended in some degree to overlook the importance of its constituent *parts*. The balance was readjusted later on by the labours of the anatomical school of Alexandria, which . . . arose in the 3rd century B.C." (in Galen, 1952, p. xii).

Six hundred years after the Hippocratic writings had been set down, Galen, that most holistic of the Hippocratic ancient physicians, was basing his practice on the Hippocratic tradition, and he too encountered opposition to his ideas. Brock has summarized his contributions to medical thought; it is interesting to note how similar some of his ideas are to current holistic thought:

> His keen appreciation of the unity of the organism, and of the inter-dependence of its parts; his realization that the vital phenomena (physiological and pathological) in a living organism can only be understood when considered in relation to the *environment* of that organism or part. . . .
>
> His realization of the inappropriateness and inadequacy of physical formulae in explaining physiological activities. . . .
>
> His clear realisation that . . . a view of the whole . . . could never be obtained by a mere summation of partial views. . . . (in Galen, 1952, pp. xxxix–xl)

The language, of course, is Brock's, and, it is reasonable to assume that his interpretation of Galen was influenced by Hegel's theory of internal relations, which will be discussed shortly. Nevertheless, Galen's own words reflect similar notions. On the relationship of body and mind, he says: "Since feeling and voluntary motion are peculiar to animals, whilst growth and nutrition are common to plants as well, we may look on the former as effects of the *soul* and the latter as effects of the *nature*. . . . And we say that animals are governed at once by their soul and by their nature" (p. 3). On the integrity of the organism and its powers of self-healing, he writes: "Nature is a constructive artist and . . . the substance of things is always tending towards unity and also towards alteration because its own parts act upon and are acted upon by one another. . . . This constructive nature has powers which attract appropriate and expel alien matter. For in no other way could she be constructive, preservative of the animal, and eliminative of its diseases" (p. 73).

Galen's views did not enjoy universal acceptance. Several medical schools of the time held conflicting theories. Among the most prominent of Galen's opponents were the followers of Asclepiades (1st century B.C.), who advocated a mechanistic system. Galen spent considerable energy trying to refute their work. It seems he largely prevailed and that his views on medicine were highly influential over the next thousand years, thus giving some credence to the claim that holistic thought in medicine was the rule before the advent of the Enlightenment.

Many figures of the period, such as Galileo, Baron, and Kepler, were instrumental in creating the revolution that paved the way to modern science. But perhaps the course of medicine and biology was most affected by Descartes (1596–1650). Certainly, germ theory as formulated by Pasteur and Koch owes a great deal to him. Physicians were freed to examine the workings of the body, once Descartes' dualism had made it their proper field for study, assigning the soul to the Church. According to Miller:

Descartes bequeathed science an awkward philosophical problem by making this distinction, but it nevertheless had certain advantages. By locking the conscious mind in a metaphysical penthouse, he made it possible to consider a large part of the human repertoire in a mechanical fashion. (1982, p. 304)

Depending upon one's point of view, therefore, Descartes either stimulated the advance of technical, scientific medicine, or hindered the further evolution of a natural, organic medicine. What he clearly did not do was extinguish the latter altogether. For example, fewer than a hundred years after the death of Descartes, La Mettrie (1709–51), a French physician, observed that mental status was not stable, but was related to the severity of bodily illness. He concluded that the life of the mind was not independent of the rest of the organism and thus was led to deny Cartesian dualism (Magner, 1979, pp. 306–307). La Mettrie's contemporary and fellow physician Jerome Gaub believed the mind and body were so closely related that "wherever there is mind there is body, and wherever body, mind" (in Rather, 1965, p. 34). He warned that, "should the physician devote all of his efforts to the body alone, and take no account of the mind, his curative endeavors will pretty often be less than happy" (p. 70). It is evident that the dualism of the eighteenth century was not absolute.

The debate carried over to the next century. The nature of conventional medicine in the United States from about 1780 to 1850 caused that period to be characterized as the "Age of Heroic Medicine." Few treatments of real efficacy were known, and patients were subjected to measures that were extremely harsh (thus heroic), probably useless, and often dangerous. Bleeding was commonplace, as was the use of drugs that caused vomiting, purging, and profuse perspiration. Local irritants were used to cause blistering of the skin (Weil, 1983).

It is little wonder that this type of treatment was regarded with horror by many observers. As patients sought health care that was less threatening than that offered by the conventional practitioners of the time, competing therapeutic systems arose to offer alternatives. The new sects, which tended to espouse less violent therapies than those prescribed by the M.D.'s, often viewed their regimens as more "natural" than those of orthodox medicine. Some, such as the Christian Scientists, believed that healing came from God, and other, nonreligious, sects tended to regard healing as a natural power of the body. Adherents of sects sometimes rejected not only heroic therapies, but also the authority of physicians as healers. Some sects substituted other healers in their stead. This was true of chiropractic, which sought legal status for its practitioners comparable to that enjoyed by M.D.'s. Others relied on individuals to act as their own physicians believing that health was attainable through such means as special diets, physical therapies, or mental maneuvers.

In spite of the fact that these alternative systems decried the practice of orthodox medicine, they were not necessarily more "holistic" in nature. As Wallis and Morley (1976) point out, both chiropractic and osteopathy can be considered more mechanistic in nature than conventional medicine, relying, as they do, on simple mechanical explanations of all diseases. Nevertheless, the alternative therapeutic systems in the first half of the nineteenth century stimulated many ideas about health and health care that would be both familiar to and admired by today's holists.

Homeopathy provides a case in point. Begun by German physician Samuel Hahnemann, it was based on the

notion that diseases could be cured by the administration
of small amounts of medication that produced symptoms
similar to those of the illness. Doses were minute because
Hahnemann claimed that medication became more po-
tent as its concentration was diluted. Homeopathy was
introduced to America early in the nineteenth century,
and had won a significant following by mid-century. Several parallels can be drawn between Kett's (1968) observations regarding the homeopathy of the last century and
the holism of the 1980s. He notes that homeopathy was
compatible with perfectionist thinking, including the
idea that robust health is the natural state of the human
organism. Referring to another alternative sect that pre-
ceded homeopathy, he contends: "To a certain extent
homeopathy appealed to the same type of person attracted by Thomsonianism—perfectionists, faddists, and
reformers" (p. 155).

Today it might be said that holism appeals to the same
type of person attracted by homeopathy. Another similarity is seen in the belief of both groups in the natural
healing powers of the body. Both seek therapies that will
foster these powers. Finally, the relationship of mind and
body is a significant issue in both holistic and homeo-
pathic thought. Hahnemann talked of a "vital force" that
was spiritual in nature, but could be manifested mate-
rially as well. Like the holists, homeopaths were more
inclined to discuss spirituality than religion. And, like
holism, "the way in which homeopathy dealt with the
relationship of matter and spirit is at once its most confusing and important aspect" (Kett, p. 141).

The alternative sects engaged in a fierce struggle for
legitimacy. During the Age of Heroic Medicine, they had
obvious appeal to the public. Even after mid-century,
when orthodox medicine began to abandon purging and
bleeding in favor of other treatments, alternative thera-

pies remained popular and new sects emerged. These sects posed a serious challenge to conventional practitioners both financially, by competing for patients, and philosophically, by casting doubt on orthodox medicine's claim to a superior understanding of the nature of disease and its treatment. Physicians of the Progressive Era (1900–17) sought to discredit sects in the eyes of the public and to establish themselves as the sole legitimate practitioners of medicine. Their eventual dominance was achieved largely through legislation and court decisions that upheld the rights of physician-dominated licensing and examining boards to define and thereby control the practice of medicine (Burrow, 1977).

The decline of sectarian medicine was not accompanied by the disappearance of all ideas advocated by the sects. Whorton (1982) has observed the continuity of several important themes advanced by health reformers in both the nineteenth and twentieth centuries, including a suspicion of conventional medicine paired with a confidence in the healing powers of nature, a belief that stress is a significant factor in many physical illnesses, and an understanding of health as more than the absence of disease. These themes and others vetted by today's holists have not been claimed exclusively by sectarians and reformers. Evidence exists that questions of organic unity, in particular, were much discussed by conventional practitioners of the nineteenth century. Florence Nightingale—certainly no sectarian—had this to say:

I remember (in my own case) a nosegay of wild flowers being sent me, and from that moment recovery becoming more rapid. People say the effect is only on the mind. It is no such thing. The effect is on the body, too. Little as we know about the way in which we are affected by form, by color, and light, we do know this, that they have an

actual physical effect. . . . Volumes are now being written and spoken upon the effect of the mind upon the
body. Much of it is true. But I wish a little more was
thought of the effect of the body on the mind. (1974,
p. 34)

Not only modern holists overlook the fact that some
"holistic" ideas are part of the heritage of the conventional health professions. Conventional providers themselves are sometimes unaware of this fact. Kozier and
Erb (1979) state: "Modern nursing care also includes a
holistic focus. Today's nurse deals with patients as emotional and social beings as well as physical beings. Care
is provided not just for a particular disease or wound but
for the health of the whole body" (pp. 13–14).

Modern nursing? Today's nurse? Are we to assume
that the nurse of several years or decades ago cared only
for injured parts and diseased systems? The literature
does not support such a conclusion. Nurses have long
used what is now being called a holistic approach. One
is struck by the similarity of descriptions of this kind of
approach written by nurses over the past four decades:

Every ill person is experiencing *both* physiologic and psy-
chologic imbalances. Physiologic imbalances create an
emotional disequilibrium and emotional imbalances
cause physiologic disturbances. Physiologic and psy-
chologic needs must be considered together if nursing
care is to be successful. (Luckmann and Sorensen, 1980,
p. 23)

Whatever its nature, illness is the consequence of the
interaction of multiple factors—the susceptible host, the
etiological agent(s), and the environment. Disturbances
at any level of organization—biochemical, cellular, sys-

temic, psychological, interpersonal, or social—are likely
to result in disturbances at other levels. (Beland, 1970,
p. 1)

The nurse's appreciation of the feelings of individual patients who go through a sequence of events in
illness . . . is judged equally important as knowledge of
pathologic changes taking place and physical nursing
needs that must be met. (Shafer, Sawyer, McCluskey,
and Beck, 1961, p. vii)

This concept of the nurse as a substitute for what the
patient lacks to make him "complete," "whole," or "independent," be the lack physical strength, will, or
knowledge, may seem limited to some who read this.
The more one thinks about it, however, the more complex the nurse's function as so defined is seen to be.
Think how rarely one sees independence, completeness,
or wholeness of mind and body! (Harmer and Henderson, 1955, p. 5)

In recent years nursing has focused more and more on
the promotion and conservation of health and the prevention of disease; the protection and care of peoples'
environment, both social and physical; and the care of
the whole patient, mind as well as body. We have seen
an increasing emphasis on the nursing of the family and
community as well as the individual and the use of education as a means of both prevention and cure. (Dock and
Stewart, 1938, p. 355)

This last quotation is particularly telling, for it could
serve as well as any recent description of holistic health
care.

Although today's holists, then, can claim neither au-
thorship nor ownership of "holistic" ideas, some truth
prevails in their claim that conventional practitioners
have neglected them in favor of a more mechanistic

("medical model") approach to healing. Wallis and Morley (1976) have pointed out that the major achievements of orthodox medicine have been in the treatment of physical disorders, leaving marginal groups to be "concerned primarily with psychosomatic and psychological disability, or problems of interpersonal relationships" (p. 16). Thus, the holists have championed the "mind" half of the mind-body equation.

Still, in conventional health care today, we see both mechanistic and holistic approaches being touted. The issue is no longer dualism vs. integration. It is accepted that mind and body have a complex relationship. Rather, the issue is one of methodology. What is the best way to study and treat this intricate organism? Can one learn about it by examining its parts and functions, or must we regard it as a whole, in relation to its environment? The argument begun so long ago has been refined, yet it continues. Modern holistic medicine does not represent a new paradigm. It is simply the latest manifestation of an old one.

Philosophy

Descartes, then, did not single-handedly usher in an era of dualism that replaced an era of universal and unchallenged holism. Philosophers before and after him have represented both notions in varying degrees. Any philosopher who addresses the nature of man must in some way engage the problem of the body and the "other." The problem is a complex one, and simple answers do not satisfy.

Plato is particularly interesting in that he seems to have

represented both arguments in different Socratic dia-
logues. Russell (1945) describes him as a dualist who
makes a clear distinction between soul and body and
quotes from the *Phaedo*:

> It has been proved to us by experience that if we would
> have true knowledge of anything we must be quit of the
> body—the soul in herself must behold things in them-
> selves: and then we shall attain the wisdom which we
> desire, and of which we say we are lovers; not while we
> live, but after death: for if while in company with the
> body the soul cannot have pure knowledge, knowledge
> must be attained after death, if at all. And thus having
> got rid of the foolishness of the body we shall be pure
> and have converse with the pure. . . . And what is pu-
> rification but the separation of the soul from the
> body? . . . And this separation and release of the soul
> from the body is termed death. (pp. 137–138)

Thus Plato suggests that, while a person lives, his soul
is necessarily but unfortunately tied to his body, which
is a hindrance in the attainment of the worthiest goal:
pure (disembodied) knowledge.

In the *Charmides*, however, he views the mind-body
connection as benign and even positive. Disregarding the
relationship can have serious consequences. The Platonic
Socrates relates to a patient the lesson he learned from
a Thracian physician:

> And again it would be very foolish to suppose that one
> could ever treat the head by itself without treating the
> whole body . . . just as one should not attempt to cure
> the eyes apart from the head, nor the head apart from
> the body, so one should not attempt to cure the body
> apart from the soul. And this . . . is the very reason why

most diseases are beyond the Greek doctors, that they
do not pay attention to the whole as they ought to do,
since if the whole is not in good condition, it is impossible
that the part should be. . . . Because nowadays . . . this
is the mistake some doctors make with their patients.
They try to produce health of the body apart from health
of the soul. (Plato, 1973, pp. 61–63)

This dialogue, written some 2,400 years ago, is star-
tling in its similarity to what is being written by today's
holistic health advocates. Plato clearly saw a connection
between the soul and body, but appears to have been
ambivalent about the purpose it served. On one occasion, he fretted that the "foolishness" of the body in-
terfered with the purposes of the soul, and on another
he pointed out that one must acknowledge and attend
to the soul in order to enhance the welfare of the body.
During life, it seems, man experiences a kind of functional unity; after death the soul is free to manifest its
free and independent nature.

Aristotle, too, struggled to explain the observations that
indicated an association between cognitive and physical
functions. Like Plato, he had difficulty reconciling three
apparently conflicting assumptions. The first is that man
is an integrated being, the second is that he is subject to
physical decay and death, and the third is that some part
of him is indestructible.

If man is a unity, then he must be altogether mortal
or entirely immortal; it is a contradiction to suggest that
he can be partly each. Plato resolved this contradiction
by suggesting that different rules hold following death.
Aristotle had more difficulty in reconciling the three assumptions. In *De Anima* he initially states very clearly:
"Thus we should not ask whether soul and body are one,

just as we should not ask whether the imprint and the wax, or a particular thing and its matter, are one; for of all the meanings of 'unity' and 'being' actuality is the primary one" (1961, p. 211). But, almost immediately after making this statement, he begins to hedge and qualify:

> Clearly, then, the soul is not separable from the body, or certain parts of it (if it can be divided into parts) are not separable; for the activity of *some* parts belongs to the parts of the body themselves. Yet *some* parts may be separable, because they are not actualizations of any body. But it is still uncertain whether the soul is the actualization of the body in the way we have discussed, or is related to it as a sailor is to his ship. (p. 212)

In his *Metaphysics* (1979), Aristotle says with more confidence: "It belongs to the physicist to investigate even some part of the soul, namely, that which does not exist without matter" (p. 103). Thus, he creates a model of man in which there is a body, and a soul that has both corporeal and noncorporeal features. The corporeal soul is responsible for integrative functions.

The ancient Greeks, of course, did not lay to rest the mind-body problem. It has continued to vex thinkers through the centuries. The two modern philosophers who have had the strongest influence on holistic thought represent opposite extremes of the holism-dualism continuum. Descartes, who has already been discussed, was father to the school of thought that advocated strict dualism, a mechanistic view of life, and an analytic approach to its study. He became a target for the holists, and the contrasts between his thinking and theirs has been used repeatedly to illuminate their ideas.

Hegel on the other hand, though he did not address the mind-body question directly, is the direct source of much modern holism. Phillips (1971, p. 3) states that several important holistic theses are based on Hegel's principle of internal relations. Among these are the assumptions that a part cannot be understood in isolation from the whole and that all parts of the whole are dynamically interrelated.

In *Science of Logic* (1929), Hegel claims that every whole consists of parts which, if viewed in isolation from the larger whole, themselves become wholes. The same progression obtains upward from parts to wholes, so that eventually this logic is forced to assert that all things stand in relation to all other things. "The infinity of the progress which results is the impossibility of combining the two ideas which the mediation contains, namely, that each of the two determinations passes over through its independence and separation from the other into dependence and into the other" (p. 148).

The point of this turgid passage seems to be that we cannot have knowledge of a thing unless we have knowledge of the larger thing of which it is a part. The difficulty comes when we realize that the larger thing is subsumed into yet another, and so on, ad infinitum. Or, as William James sarcastically commented on Hegel: "The full truth about anything involves more than that thing. In the end nothing less than the whole of everything can be the truth of anything at all" (1977, p. 513). This Hegelian grandeur is reflected in the sweeping statements of some of today's holists about man's relationship to the universe.

Other key ideas of modern holism were formulated by philosophers of the nineteenth century who were markedly influenced by Hegel. Phillips (1976) lists five interrelated ideas that these thinkers used when discussing organic wholes.

1. The analytic approach as typified by the physico-chemical sciences proves inadequate when applied to certain cases—for example, to a biological organism, to society, or even to reality as a whole.
2. The whole is more than the sum of its parts.
3. The whole determines the nature of its parts.
4. The parts cannot be understood if considered in isolation from the whole.
5. The parts are dynamically interrelated or interdependent. (p. 6)

All these theses can be traced to Hegel and his followers. Every modern holist subscribes to at least some of them—a tribute to their enduring attraction.

William James was well aware of the power these ideas had to command attention. He admitted to it when he said: "There is no doubt that most of us find that the bare notion of an absolute all-one is inspiring. 'I yielded myself to the perfect whole,' writes Emerson; and where can you find a more mind-dilating object? A certain loyalty is called forth by the idea; even if not proved actual, it must be believed in somehow. Only an enemy of philosophy can speak lightly of it" (1977, p. 500).

But, although he acknowledged the possibility that unity and connection *may* exist in the universe, he opposed Hegel's *assumption* that it did. And he was merciless with those who tried to foist this assumption on others as obvious fact: "When a young man first conceives the notion that the whole world forms one great fact . . . he feels as if he were enjoying a great insight,

and looks superciliously on all who still fall short of this
sublime conception" (1974, p. 91).

James sought to reconcile the seemingly contradictory
notions of unity and unrelatedness in the universe. He
refused to follow the Hegelians in their leap from the
observation that some things are related to the assumption that all things are related:

> Radical empiricism and pluralism stand out for the legiti-
> macy of the notion of *some*: each part of the world is in
> some ways connected, in some other ways not connected
> with its other parts, and the ways can be discriminated,
> for many of them are obvious, and their differences are
> obvious to view. (1977, p. 510)

> [Pragmatism] must equally abjure absolute monism and
> absolute pluralism. The world is One just so far as its
> parts hang together by any definite connexion. It is many
> just so far as any definite connexion fails to obtain. And
> finally it is growing more and more unified by those sys-
> tems of connexion at least which human energy keeps
> framing as time goes on. (1974, p. 105)

James is so eminently reasonable regarding the issue
of monism, so generous in acknowledging its virtues, so
careful and clear in discussing its faults, that one must
wonder why his work has not had stronger influence on
today's holists. He is rarely referred to in their papers;
indeed, he seems to have been largely overlooked by
them. When he is cited, it is usually in reference to his
later, more mystical works, such as *The Varieties of Religious Experience*. How is it that the rest of his writings
has been ignored? It seems likely that, among the more
orthodox holists, his view of the partial and incomplete
connections in the universe is unacceptably lukewarm.

It does not support their more expansive ideas. It stops where they begin. James was unwilling to go further than saying that some things are connected, whereas the holists began by noting that some things are connected, and proceeded to solder the entire universe together.

A more charitable and equally likely reason for James's lack of standing among the holists is the cosmological nature of his work. In much of it, he does not address the question of the mind-body connection directly and hence he was of less interest to those who stood opposed to dualism. Those in health care, particularly, turn to thinkers who consider the nature of man rather than the nature of the universe.

Yet, this can be only a partial explanation of James's faint influence on the holists. Hegel, after all, also spoke about the universe. But his monism fitted perfectly with holistic thought. James's pluralism, though it accommodated the connections apparent in nature, did not. It may be that the holists have tiptoed around James because he had pointed out the gaps in their perfectly constructed universe.

Psychology

John Dewey has said, "There was a time when philosophy, science and the arts, medicine included, were much closer together than they have been since" (1968, p. 299). The disciplines have become more distinct. Still, it is difficult to determine the point at which philosophy and psychology diverge. Although Dewey is certainly numbered among the major American philosophers, I have chosen to begin the discussion of the contributions of psychology to holistic thought with him. While both James and Dewey were functionalists, Dewey's 1896 paper "The Reflex Arc Concept in Psychology" is commonly regarded as having been the basis of functional psychology (Phillips, 1976, p. 114).

With Dewey's work, for the first time, one begins to discern a fairly clear line of development beginning with the functionalist and Gestalt psychologies leading to the organismic psychologies, and finally to humanistic psychology, from which the holistic health movement drew so heavily. Yet, in the intervening years, little has been said about holistic man and holistic health that Dewey did not say himself. Some of his thoughts, in fact, were merely affirmations of Hegelian theses. He claimed, for example, that an organic whole cannot be understood by examining its parts: "We may isolate a particular organic structure or process for study . . . but we cannot understand the organism until we have taken its history into account" (1968, p. 308).

He vigorously rejected dualism and believed that the artificial separation of mind and body was responsible for many of the problems encountered in the practice of medicine. In "The Unity of the Human Being" (1939), he addressed a group of physicians on the subject. Urging them to abandon dualism, he stated that "we cannot be scientific save as we seek for the physiological, the physical factor in every emotional, intellectual and volitional experience. . . . And it is also true that our knowledge of social relations and their effects upon native and original physiological processes is scanty and unorganized in comparison with the physical knowledge at command" (pp. 827–828).

Just as holistic practitioners do today, Dewey suggested that the health of individuals is affected by their relations to others as well as to the environment and urged that more attention be given to preventive medicine. And, just like today's holists, he thought he saw a "paradigm shift" occurring:

> The consequences of this divided education are writ large in the state of our civilization. The physician meets them in a wide range of induced disorders, to say nothing of waste and incapacitation. The walls which mark the separation are beginning to crack, although they are far from crumbling. From all sides the artificiality of isolation from one another of mind and body are commencing to be seen. There is at least the beginning of co-operation between those who are traditionally occupied with the concerns of mind and those busy with the affairs of the body. (1968, p. 316)

Thus did Dewey anticipate many of the ideas of today's "new" paradigm.

The German Gestalt psychologists Wertheimer, Kohler, and Koffka, active also during the early 1900s, conceived a psychology that in some ways was compatible with Dewey's and that also influenced the holistic health movement. According to advocates of Gestalt theory, the human organism perceives and responds to whole percepts of events or interactions, not merely to discrete stimuli. Using concepts formulated by European phenomenologists, Gestalt theory disavows clear distinctions between sensation and perception, perception and cognition, and the dualism implied by those distinctions (Misiak and Sexton, 1973, p. 57).

Kurt Goldstein's work was strongly influenced by Gestalt theory (Shaffer, 1978). Trained in neurology and psychiatry, Goldstein worked extensively with brain-injured soldiers during World War I. His clinical observation of many of them contributed to his organismic theory (Hall and Lindzey, 1970). Like the Hegelians, Goldstein believed that the whole is more than the sum of its parts, and that the parts cannot be understood if considered in isolation, though he did concede a place for analysis if the organic whole were kept in mind:

> Yet ultimately our procedure is rooted in a more profound conviction: this is *the conviction that a state of greater perfection can never be understood from that of less perfection, and that only the converse is possible.* It is very feasible to isolate parts from a whole, but a perfect whole can never be composed by synthesizing it from the less perfect parts. (1939, p. 515)

And, like Dewey, he regarded the human organism as an indivisible unit:

> Neither does the mind act on the body, nor the body on the mind, no matter how much this may seem to be the case in superficial observation. We are always dealing with the activity of the whole organism, the effects of which we refer at one time to something called mind, at another time to something called body. . . . We . . . demand that the psychological and the physical should be treated as phenomena which have to be evaluated as to their significance for the holistic reality of the organism, in the situation in which we observe it. (p. 340)

Perhaps Goldstein's most original contribution to psychology was the concept of self-actualization. This he defined as the tendency of an organism to behave in such a way as to realize its potential. No drives exist save self-actualization, and what we call "needs" are merely forms of the one need to self-actualize:

> What are usually called drives are tendencies correspond-ing to the capacities, the nature of the organism, and the environment in which the organism is living at a given time. It is better that we speak of "needs." The organism has definite potentialities, and because it has them it has the need to actualize or realize them. The fulfillment of these needs represents the self-actualization of the or-ganism. (p. 204)

Goldstein felt that, when an organism is behaving in a way that seems to interfere with its actualization, it is because the conditions for realization of its capacities are unfavorable. His concept of human nature as an organic entity that will fulfill itself given the right circumstances was a key concept in the thinking of the humanistic psy-chologists.

Abraham Maslow—a colleague of Goldstein's at Bran-deis University who is widely regarded as the father of humanistic psychology—acknowledged his debt to Goldstein by dedicating his book *Toward a Psychology of Being* to him (1968). Interestingly, it is Maslow and not Goldstein who has become most identified with the con-cept of self-actualization. Maslow described his use of the term in this way:

> The term, first coined by Kurt Goldstein, is being used in this book in a much more specific and limited fashion. It refers to man's desire for self-fulfillment, namely, to the tendency for him to become actualized in what he is potentially. This tendency might be phrased as the desire to become more and more what one idiosyncratically is,

to become everything that one is capable of becoming. (1970, p. 46)

This notion of human potential is of key importance in Maslow's work and is apparent (as is Goldstein's influence) in some of the assumptions he makes about human nature:

> We have, each of us, an essential biologically based inner nature. . . .
> This inner nature, as much as we know of it so far, seems not to be intrinsically . . . evil. . . .
> Since this inner nature is good or neutral rather than bad, it is best to bring it out and to encourage it rather than to suppress it. . . .
> If this essential core of the person is denied or suppressed, he gets sick. . . . (1968, pp. 3–4)

One of Maslow's best-known ideas, the hierarchy of needs, was based on Goldstein's assertion that needs, not drives, form the basis of behavior and that they derive from the larger need for self-actualization. Maslow describes a two-part hierarchy consisting of basic needs and growth needs. Only if the basic needs for physical requirements, safety and security, love and belongingness, and esteem are met can one attend to the growth needs, which include such things as goodness, simplicity, and meaningfulness. It is a mark of self-actualized persons that they are able to meet many of their growth needs (1968, 1970, 1971).

Maslow proposed that the most fruitful way to learn about how people fulfill the potential of their inner selves is to study individuals who are already most fully self-actualized. His belief that an understanding of health could not issue from observation of disease led him to investigate those persons—both living and historical figures—who represented to him successful self-actualization. He found them to be creative, spontaneous, autonomous individuals who related to themselves and others in an accepting, nonstereotyped manner. They demonstrated a certain detachment and had a larger than average need for privacy (1970).

Such self-actualizers, however, represent the exception rather than the rule. Most of us muddle along worrying about our basic needs. And even high actualizers are only relatively actualized; they move closer to or further from the ideal as they make choices in living. Maslow sees self-actualization as a process, not an achievement.

But all of us, he says, experience movements of self-actualization called peak experiences that are " . . . transient . . . moments of ecstasy which cannot be bought, cannot be guaranteed, cannot even be sought" (1971, p. 48). These experiences have a transcendent, mystical quality during which the person feels more integrated, whole, one with the world, and fully aware and functioning (1968, pp. 103–114).

The tremendous impact of Maslow's work on the holistic health movement has been widely acknowledged; his name is to be found in the bibliographies of many holistic books and articles. The Maslowian concepts of man's nature as essentially good or neutral, growth and fulfillment as the natural course of development, self-actualization, hierarchy of needs, and peak experiences have found their way repeatedly into the holistic literature and have been embraced by holistic practitioners. I think I do not state the case too strongly when I suggest that Maslow and the other humanistic psychologists (notably Rogers) provided the theoretical framework for much of the holistic health movement.

Counterculture and the Human Potential Movement

The link between humanistic psychology and holistic health is clear, but not direct. A detour occurred in the late 1960s and the 1970s through the counterculture and the human potential movement (Berliner and Salmon, 1980). These movements grew up together. Although they were distinct, they had much in common; many people found them virtually indistinguishable. Shaffer (1978) points out that the counterculture shared several values with humanistic psychology, including a sense of "rebellion against an alienating society," "the rejection of the idea of role-appropriate behavior," "the need to expand one's consciousness," and "an avoidance of the Western tendency to view polarities in a dichotomous, either-or fashion . . . in favor of more Eastern, Zen-like conceptions of polarity" (pp. 8–9). It is not surprising that humanistic thought was congenially received by the counterculture.

Maslow's influence is clearly seen in the term "human potential," which suggests the self-actualizing tendency of the human organism. The notion that people are capable of change and growth throughout their lives and ought to be encouraged to exercise their potential for growth has been an article of faith in the human potential movement.

Carl Rogers, perhaps, provided the most direct link between those in conventional psychology and those in

the human potential movement with his work in encounter groups. Although Lewin and others had been
conducting T-groups since 1946 (Schloss, Siroka, and
Siroka, 1971), Rogers (1970) was a pioneer in the use of
such groups for the purpose of personal growth.

Humanistic psychology has much in common with the
holistic health movement as well. Shaffer cites the following as central emphases of humanistic psychology.

1. Humanism is strongly phenomenological or experi-
   ential: its starting point is conscious experience.
2. Humanistic psychology insists on man's essential
   wholeness and integrity.
3. Humanistic psychology, while acknowledging that
   there are clear-cut limits inherent in human existence, insists that human beings retain an essential
   freedom and autonomy.
4. Humanistic psychology is antireductionistic in its orientation.
5. Humanistic psychology, consistent with its strong
   grounding in existentialism, believes that human nature can never be fully defined. (1978, pp. 10–17)

Each of these ideas, echoing Hegel, Goldstein, and
Maslow, found its way into the philosophy of holistic
health. In the late sixties and early seventies, holistic
health had not yet emerged as a distinct entity. Yet, interest was growing in the health of the body as part of
total health, or self-actualization. In the human potential
movement, this was manifested in various therapies,
known collectively as bodywork, which attempted to foster health by achieving integration and balance within
the person (Capra, 1982).

The counterculture was attracted to health and healing. Members were particularly intrigued with the exotic,

the ancient, and the non-Western. Almost anything was worth investigating so long as it did not represent conventional Western medicine, which was considered highly suspect. In part, this was a reflection of the counterculture's rejection of authority of all kinds as well as the physical and natural sciences in particular. In his book *The Making of a Counter-Culture*, Theodore Roszak questioned the legitimacy of the authority claimed by health professionals:

> If we are cured of disease, we explain the matter by saying a pill or a serum did it—as if that were to say anything at all. . . . We believe that somewhere behind the pills . . . there are experts who understand whatever else there is to understand. We know they are experts, because, after all, they talk like experts and besides possess degrees, licenses, titles, and certificates. Are we any better off than the savage who believes his fever has been cured because an evil spirit has been driven out of his system? (1969, p. 259)

The counterculture sought health care that was compatible with its belief system and found itself attracted to non- or pre-professional types of healing. Interest was strong in anything "natural," be it food, environment, or medicine.

People began to investigate the healing systems of primitive societies, and interest in primitive medicine is still very much in evidence in today's holistic health movement. Flynn (1980) writes that "in primitive times, men and women believed that disease was caused by spiritual powers which must be fought by spiritual means. . . . This view of illness, still prevalent in current primitive cultures, makes use of the will to health and the power of suggestion in a holistic attitude which deals with the whole person in their environment" (p. 41).

Foster and Anderson (1978) propose two categories of primitive medical systems: naturalistic and personalistic. In the first of these, disease is believed to be caused by an imbalance within the individual or between the individual and his environment. Any disturbance in equilibrium can lead to disease. Practitioners of Indian Ayurvedic medicine, for example, believe that the body has three humours, or *dosha*. For a person to enjoy good health, the dosha must be maintained in harmony. Certain foods, for instance, can alter the balance among the dosha.

Personalistic systems, on the other hand, are not predicated on an equilibrium model. In these systems, disease is believed to result from the deliberate intent of an agent. The agent may be a human being possessing special powers, such as a witch, or it may be a god, ghost, ancestor or other nonhuman. Ritual behavior is often used to protect an individual from the influence of such an agent, as is the case with the Gadsup people of New Guinea, who place ashes on the foreheads of newborns to protect them from evil spirits (Leininger, 1978).

Both naturalistic and personalistic medical systems had strong appeal within the counterculture. Classical Chinese medicine, which was based on a naturalistic philosophy, was held in especially high regard. In classical Chinese medicine, the Tao, or The Way, is that power which created the universe and the five elements of fire, water, wood, metal, and earth. It also created and continues to control the complementary forces of Yin and Yang. The Tao maintains the balance of Yin and Yang necessary to preserve order in the universe. Man is required to live by the natural laws of the Tao, or he risks illness. According to Veith, the ancient Chinese believed that "man, who was created with the universe and in its image, owed his health and hence his life to the harmony of natural forces; if this harmony was upset, the result was disease and death. But while the macrocosm of the universe was left to the course of Tao and the natural forces, it was up to man to shape his fate by compliance with Tao, the Way, and thus to keep the proper balance of Yin and Yang, the two opposing forces" (1973, p. 17).

Those ideas appealed to those in the sixties and seventies who were striving to live in harmony with the laws of nature. Quite possibly they created a heightened interest in environmental concerns. Most certainly they influenced the holistic health movement. Participants in the counterculture borrowed several concepts from the Chinese, including the belief that health is the product of balance—within the person, and between the person and the forces of the universe, and the related belief that individuals, by choosing to live in harmony with the laws of nature, may avoid illness and are thus responsible for their own health. Along with these beliefs, the Chinese held that the prevention of illness, not the treatment of illness, was the most worthy activity of a physician (Bridgman, 1974). This idea too, was adopted by the counterculture.

Personalistic systems were also investigated. Foster and Anderson note that these systems often include shamanistic healers who possess special powers to mediate between the sick person and the disease-causing spirit. Shamanistic healing is, therefore, spiritual healing, and as such is consonant with the body-mind-spirit orientation of holistic health. According to Mattson, "advocates sometimes draw parallels between shamans and holistic healers and extol the wisdom of the shamans" (1982, p. 112).

Other traditional healers, such as *curanderos* and herbalists, also found favor within the counterculture. They were regarded as more attuned to the cultural, psychological, and spiritual determinants of health than were conventional practitioners, and were believed to be effective in cases that resisted the efforts of Western medicine. According to Foster and Anderson (1978):

> The stereotypical picture of the traditional curer is known to us all: a wise and skilled person who knows not only the patient but also the family, who is aware of the social and personal tensions of the patient's life, who sees relief from interpersonal stress as essential to relief from physical symptoms. The stereotypical curer is, in short, a social pathologist, able and willing to spend unlimited time with a single patient, little concerned with payment. (p. 249)

In fact, the anthropological literature does contain many such descriptions. Spector (1979) says that the *curandero* in Hispanic-American communities maintains a close relationship with patients and a friendly relationship with their families, will come to the house day or night, is generally less expensive than a physician, has ties to the "world of the sacred," and shares the world view of the patient (p. 257). Similarly, Kiteme (1976) states:

> African traditional doctors are experts of the mind. They are psychiatrists and psychotherapists. They have immense wisdom, sagaciousness, expertise, and knowledge regarding the African psyche, mentality, society, tradition, and social problems. They counsel on marital and personal problems, psychosomatic and organic diseases, bringing up children, and responsibilities of men and women in society. . . . In short, the traditional doc-

tors seek to create harmony between the body and the
mind and the world around us. (pp. 413–414)

The stereotypical notion of the traditional healer as
benign, effective, and attentive to the nonphysical as well
as the physical aspects of the disease was readily accepted in the counterculture, and later in the holistic
health movement. This picture was often contrasted with
a depiction of Western healers as limited in skill; narrow
in focus; excessively interested in remuneration; and at
a loss to even diagnose, much less treat, certain illnesses
that could be handled with ease by a traditional healer.
Foster and Anderson (1978), however, point out that the
stereotypical picture of the traditional healer may be in-
accurate. They refer to Press's work regarding the *curanderos* of Bogota, who may spend as few as five minutes
with a patient and then charge a high fee. Certainly the
stereotypical healers' skills seem exaggerated.

Some anthropologists have described the tendency to
glorify the traditional healer as a form of extreme cultural
relativism. Foster and Anderson quote Stein: "Anthropologists have been absolutely phobic in their contempt
for Western (read: dehumanizing) medicine. Through
our contempt of Western civilization, our patient bias,
and our transference to our favorite primitives (patients,
ethnic groups, traditional healers), we seem unable to
identify with the vilified Western medical professionals
and their institutions. . . . I am afraid it will take some
working-through before we are able to be skeptical about
shamanic-native cures" (p. 131).

The counterculture, as its name indicates, rejected
much of Western culture, including its medical system.
In doing so, it was guilty of the kind of extreme cultural
relativism Stein ascribed to anthropologists. Certainly,

traditional healers have been successful within their societies. Nevertheless, their effectiveness is limited.

These limits are recognized even by the clients who patronize them. Henderson and Primeaux (1981) describe the tendency of many Third World patients to "shop around" for health care and to use both Western and indigenous healers. They also note that many traditional curers incorporate aspects of Western medicine into their own practices. Quintanilla (1976) observes that certain Peruvian Indians, finding the Western doctor more successful in certain instances than the local healers, have concluded that some diseases are appropriately treated by Western medicine. Quintanilla believes that many of the problems deemed by the Indians as treatable by local healers are psychological in nature and attributes the greater success of local healers to their ability to communicate with patients and to use suggestion effectively.

Similarly, Moore, Van Arsdale, Glittenberg, and Aldrich (1980) suggest that traditional healers have enjoyed success with the sociopsychological aspects of cure, and that Western medicine has been particularly effective in the biomedical aspects of care. The healers themselves are likely to be aware of their limitations, and may attempt to increase their success rates by careful screening of clients, accepting only those likely to be cured (Wood, 1979). The counterculture, however, manifested a naive willingness to overlook the limitations of traditional healers and to assign to them the exaggerated characteristics described by Foster and Anderson.

Primitive medicine was but one of the systems explored by the counterculture. As was mentioned earlier, almost anything unorthodox was of interest. Many techniques, therapies, and traditions were investigated, including some that can only be characterized as bizarre.

And out of this jumble of the mystical, the traditional, the occult, the Oriental, and common sense the modern holistic health movement was born.

It has a sprawling family tree. From philosophy through the ages, it inherited an understanding of man as an integrated being—an understanding confirmed by the findings of medical science. Its more immediate fore-bears of humanistic psychology and the human potential movement provided the notion that this integrated man has great, largely untapped potential for growth. Finally, the counterculture contributed a suspicion of Western medicine, coupled with a contradictory enthusiasm for other traditions, and the conviction that health could be controlled by the individual.

It is perhaps no accident that holistic health should have emerged in the turbulent 1960s. As Whorton (1982) has observed, "Radical schemes of hygiene have been a constant feature of American life since the early 1800s, but they have naturally flourished in periods of general reformist ferment and social optimism when an expand-ing public spirit enlarged the constituency for perfec-tionist campaigns" (pp. 11–12). Certainly the sixties were a time of great hope for the possibility of change, both in the social order and in individuals. Although holistic thought has a long tradition in many disciplines, includ-ing medicine, it was the counterculture that was the di-rect antecedent of the holistic health movement.

Summary

Biological holism has been and continues to be a dev-ilishly tricky and highly debatable concept. Yet, some people consider the case closed. They proclaim rather than argue their case: man is whole, all of a piece—this simple truth is so self-evident that no other possibilities are to be considered. Maslow (1970) actually went so far as to suggest that people who fail to understand this are suffering from some sort of mental illness (one wonders how William James would respond to the following):

> Holism is obviously true—after all, the cosmos is one and interrelated; any society is one and interrelated; any person is one and interrelated, etc. . . . Recently I have become more and more inclined to think that the atomistic way of thinking is a form of mild psychopathology. (p. xi)

The legacy of uncertainty is lost; and the tradition of debate is abandoned. The infinitely complex questions about human nature that men have struggled with for thousands of years have been reduced to a series of pronouncements and formulas.

2

Holistic Health: Movement and Slogans

In this chapter, an attempt will be made to describe and define the holistic health movement. Although describing various holistic ideas is a fairly straightforward proposition, demonstrating how they have coalesced into a movement is not. Actually, though I have been using the term "movement" to designate the activities and ideas involved, it is not entirely clear that this is the appropriate term. Even the holists themselves seem confused. In the first two paragraphs of her discussion of holism, one author describes it as a set of practices, an approach, a philosophy, a movement, a system, and a model! (Brallier, 1978). Another writer contends that "we are in danger of obscuring more than we reveal when we use the term 'holistic,' which looks as if it soon will be eviscerated of any specific meaning" (Kleinman, 1981, p. 450). Read (1983) has this to say about the holists: "These 'new' medicine enthusiasts have constituted themselves informally as a 'movement,' developing a consistent terminology and a semblance of organizational structure" (p. 382).

Vanderpool (1984), on the other hand, has argued that the various groups using the term "holistic" are too diverse to be characterized as a movement: "No uniform set of holistic therapies can be identified, and no common institutions are found among its advocates. In fact, so much diversity exists among the proponents of holism that it can scarcely be considered a single movement" (p. 773). Vanderpool makes a significant point. The ideas and practices embraced by one group of holists may not be shared by another such group. Nor, as Vanderpool further notes, are such ideas and practices necessarily unique to holistic health; some belong to one of several traditions within conventional health care. Thus, he is correct in suggesting that the term "holistic health movement" is problematic.

It can be demonstrated, however, that, despite their differences, persons who identify themselves as holists share some common beliefs about health and some common goals regarding health care. Furthermore, the existence of holistic journals and organizations indicates that the theme provides a common ground for diverse groups. It is probably as valid to talk about a holistic health movement as it is to talk about a women's movement. "Movement" probably comes as close as any available term to describing the collective activity of the holists. Therefore, despite its lack of precision, it will be used in this book.

Considering the difficulty that the holists have in articulating what they are about, perhaps I may be forgiven a certain vagueness in my own use of several other terms as well. Throughout this volume, I will rely on the following loose definitions:

> *Holist*: Minimally, someone who subscribes to the thesis that an organic whole is more than the sum of its parts, and who rejects mind/body dualism.

Holistic health care: A system of health care predicated
on the above. Advocates of holistic care may agree on
these ideas and very little else. Practices range from the
exotic to the conventional; practitioners from the suspect
to those licensed as professionals.

Definitions found in the literature, though similar, are
generally vague and offer few particulars. Svihus's definition is representative:

Holistic health, then, is a state of integration of the physical body and of the mental and emotional soul-self, in
harmony with the spiritual self. . . . The concept refers
to the fact that the whole of a person is greater than the
mere sum of his parts, and that there is an approach to
the whole person who is ill, instead of merely to his parts
or to his illness as if they were separate from the whole
of him. (1979, pp. 480–481)

I believe this definition would be acceptable to a majority
of holists, and that it exemplifies the core of basic beliefs
around which the movement is organized: man is whole;
any threat to his wholeness will cause him to sicken; an
adequate health-care system must recognize and act on
these truths.

Among holists, these beliefs are considered to be plain
facts, so self-evident that they scarcely need explaining
or defending. Yet, not all their claims are obvious or consistent. It would seem fair to inquire whether or not the
empirical claim of human wholeness is valid. To this, the
holist would likely respond: "Of course! It is obvious to
see." And, on the face of it, he would be correct. A
professional baseball player uses his mind to learn the
rules of the game and to assess the possibilities as he
steps up to the plate. His body has been trained for this

activity. Yet the actual performance simultaneously engages his mind and body as he calculates the speed and trajectory of the ball even as he swings. It would be difficult to observe the smooth response of the organism to various stimuli without concluding that there was evidence of integration and wholeness.

But humans can be described in many ways, some of them equally compelling. Freud's concept of the unconscious, for example, has been wonderfully fruitful in helping us to understand and explain behavior. Its function is considered normal, yet it speaks to a lack of complete integration within the person—"part" of whom is harboring feelings and wishes that are unavailable, at least under ordinary circumstances, to the rest of the individual. Regardless of whether or not one accepts Freud's entire scheme, it is difficult to write off the concept of the subconscious altogether.

The holistic model is not so clearly superior to all others as to demand our allegiance. Nor is it always internally consistent. While extolling wholeness, holists also express admiration for Eastern meditative techniques that elicit dissociative states and use tools such as hypnosis that cause similar responses. If wholeness is the goal, why attempt to create a subjective state in which one's mind and body are experienced as detached, or in which one is only minimally aware of either? Consider the so-called "runner's high," in which a sensation of euphoria replaces the pain and exhaustion caused by strenuous exercise. Is this an example of wholeness, or is it the result of an inappropriate decision to allow the body to ignore the message of pain?

These examples raise the question of whether or not integration and wholeness are one and the same. Holists have failed to provide a satisfactory description of whole-

ness. A problem not adequately addressed is the difficulty of even talking about man without using terms like
body and mind or spirit, terms that imply parts. This
problem is roughly patched over with the use of modi-
fiers such as related, unified, integrated, synthesized,
and harmonious. Griffith says: "For man *is* a synthesis:
he is not spirit, mind and matter glued together, but a
synthesis of these things so tragically ripped apart" (in
Spicker, 1970, p. 274). Zaner (1981) notes that such a
concept was shared by Descartes himself, who believed
that the body was "intimately unioned" with the mind.
For holists, this would appear to be an attempt to have
their whole cake and the parts of it too. As Zaner points
out, "the 'union' is ultimately an abortive notion, for its
very sense effectively buys into a dualism, if only incipi-
ently" (p. 11).

Another model has been described by Hans Jonas, who
suggests that, though the organism is one, it has dual
aspects that may be experienced and apprehended. In
Zaner's words:

> There truly *is* no "union" but rather the "one" living
> body whose "extensiveness" locates it within the actual
> world. . . . The dual*ism* is wrong for it renders the dual
> aspects of reality, grounded in the dual*ity* of the orga-
> nism, into ontological substances. *Both the aspects are my-
> self.* . . . There are not two *things*, then, to be by some
> ledgerdemain welded together; there is rather the one
> and only embodied person, whose being is, however,
> *intrinsically complex, dual.* (pp. 11–12)

This argument acknowledges but does not satisfactorily
resolve the contradiction of the whole comprised of
parts.

Some confusion exists, too, about whether the claim of human wholeness is normative or prescriptive. Holists insist that it is a critical defining characteristic of the human organism. Yet, holistic health therapies are largely a compendium of practices designed to move the person *toward* wholeness. This is problematic given the definition of holists that posits wholeness as a requisite. They would argue that any sign of fragmentation is associated with illness, and therefore supports their claim that wholeness is the norm.

But it is impossible to conceive of moving toward something that we necessarily are. Some, not willing to give up the normative claim altogether, have suggested that such practices move an individual toward a "state of greater wholeness," seeming to suggest that a person can be partly whole! Others advance the more modest prescriptive version which holds that it is possible and highly desirable for people to function in a more integrated, coherent fashion than they generally do. The strength of this argument is more readily apparent in our everyday lives. Most of us can recall episodes in which we were feeling unwell—dis-integrated—because we were unaware of some conflict between physical and emotional needs, or because we chose to attend to one need at the expense of another. It has not been sufficiently demonstrated, however, that absolute integration is the most salutary state achievable. By that standard, a holy man who remains celibate and devotes his life to prayer cannot be healthy.

These are problems that those in the holistic health movement have yet to resolve or, in some cases, even articulate. They will need to be addressed if the movement is to refine the vague and contradictory notions that now make up its theoretical framework.

The Desire for Wholeness

Still, the movement cannot be written off on the basis
of the arguments given above. Although the holists may
not have stated their case plainly and convincingly, the
idea of human wholeness maintains a tremendous appeal
for most of us—one, as James has noted, that cannot be
lightly dismissed. Our experienced sense of ourselves as
whole, or at least as integrated beings, demands our attention. It would be unfair to regard it simply as a mental
fantasy without basis in fact because we live our lives
with a tacit recognition of its importance. "The logic of
all human experience tells us that we are *whole*," asserts
M. E. Levine (1971, p. 253). Our language can reflect our
admiration of and desire for a sense of unity. We respect
the person who is "together" and express a sense of
helplessness by explaining "I just fell to pieces."

Feelings of helplessness and lack of control, in fact,
underlie much of our desire for wholeness. Our lives
seem to grow increasingly complex; we feel less able all
the time to control the events in our world. We share
with Yeats the conviction that "things fall apart, the center cannot hold." This has created a strong urge toward
that which signifies wholeness and simplicity and away
from those ideas and events that threaten complexity,
disjuncture, even chaos.

Today's holists, recognizing and sharing the resultant
anxiety, have constructed a program that attempts to
meet our need for control and order. The holistic health
movement is largely a response to expressions of frustration over our failure to meet that need. It offers a system that seeks to explain, simplify, and control
phenomena related to the individual as well as to the
world at large. The basic tenet of the system is that unity

is a cardinal fact of the universe and is to be found in man as in the galaxies and in the relationship between the two. Thus, the holistic health movement is grand in scale and does not limit its concerns to man's health.

The holists, of course, are neither the first nor the only group to propose such an all-encompassing design. It is interesting to note that they have in common with the Cartesians the search for an absolute scheme capable of explaining all phenomena and a belief in the perfectibility of man and his institutions. Hausheer says of the rationalists of the Enlightenment: "What all these rationalist thinkers shared was the belief that somewhere, by some means, a single, coherent, unified structure of knowledge concerning questions of both fact and value was in principal available" (in Berlin, 1980, p. xxvi). The holists propose that, by seeking and applying the universal rules relating to wholeness, humans can become more nearly perfect. Like any universal system, this one fails to explain everything. Ambiguity and randomness remain. This fact is disconcerting to the holists, however, who sometimes respond to an unexplained event by attempting to force it into the holistic scheme, regardless of fit. Holists illuminate the faults in their own system when they pit it against the disorderly universe, insisting that it cohere.

We are left with the tension between the real need for a system that helps to explain human phenomena and the dangers and limitations of such a system. The holists point out that Western medicine has not always served us well, that it is impersonal, fragmented, and often ineffective. They claim that their system, though also imperfect, offers a better way. Out of our yearning for order, our need for coherence and intelligibility, we cannot help but respond. We fervently wish the claims to be true.

The Movement Defined: Statements and Slogans

Some holists have recognized the need to make a clearer statement of their program than has hitherto been provided by earnest but vague definitions. Authors who have tried to go beyond these fuzzy kinds of definitions have sometimes tried to describe holistic health by offering a list of beliefs or tenets to which they subscribe. A number of these have become catch-phrases of the movement and have spread beyond its confines as well. Thus, such expressions as "You are responsible for your own health" and "Health is more than the absence of disease" have become popular and are widely repeated.

Scheffler (1960) has noted a similar phenomenon in education. He calls such statements "slogans" when they represent the spirit of a movement:

> Slogans in education provide rallying symbols of the key ideas and attitudes of educational movements. They both express and foster community of spirit, attracting new adherents and providing reassurance and strength to veterans. They are thus analogous to religious and political slogans and, like these, products of the party spirit. (p. 36)

Scheffler states that slogans are often derived from a more fully and carefully constructed theory. They themselves are not theory, but mere fragments, intended to engage our imaginations. Holistic health, however, has yet to establish its theory and is in a sense working backward by beginning with a series of slogan-like statements. Slogans, as Scheffler points out, can serve a useful purpose, but they cannot substitute for a well-developed and clearly expressed statement of the basic ideas of a movement. Nor can they even be strung together to form a definition of the primary concept—holism—though they are sometimes used as definitions. The holistic health movement, lacking a theoretical framework, or even a definition of its basic concept, relies on its slogans, which provide but a frail foundation.

Scheffler claims that slogans, which are originally merely symbols of a movement, come to be interpreted more literally as time goes on. This may be particularly likely in the case of holistic slogans, which do not so much represent the thinking of the movement as they are the concrete statements of it. They serve a twofold purpose, acting both as slogan and as theory: they attempt to be explanatory as well as evocative. Thus, a statement such as "A good practitioner must care for the whole person" comes to be understood in a more literal way than perhaps was originally intended. When this is the case, Scheffler contends, a dual evaluation of the statement is justified and called for. The statement ought to be examined as a literal statement of fact (Is it possible to care for the whole person?) and in terms of its practical purport in the context in which it is being used. Therefore, in this example, we would consider the possibility that what is being suggested is that the person being cared for be regarded as something more than a disease.

The remainder of this chapter will examine the statements used by holists to describe and define their movement. Although they are far from reaching universal agreement as to basic tenets, the following statements are frequently cited and characterize the mainstream of the movement. Each of them will be discussed briefly from the holistic point of view, and the current usage will be described. A fuller evaluation of the literal accuracy and practical use of these statements will be presented in the following chapters.

The Individual

1. *THE PERSON, LIKE ANY ORGANIC WHOLE, IS MORE THAN THE SUM OF HIS PARTS.* This claim has been borrowed from Hegel's theory of internal relations and modified by the holists to apply to man. Essentially, it is an argument against reductionism in medicine. Man, they claim, cannot be understood as an assortment of organs or functions that, when viewed collectively, constitutes a person. Rather, he must be recognized as a whole being whose unique self could not possibly be imagined from his components.

Modern medicine is accused of failing to acknowledge this fact, and the result is that patients are treated as cases, diseases, symptoms, or problems. This kind of care is regarded as de-humanizing: the client is being considered as a thing, not a person. The holists suggest that such treatment is unlikely to effect a cure.

Conventional practitioners within the movement, especially doctors, however, are quick to point out that reductionism in the form of the scientific method has allowed medicine to make major advances in the care of the sick (LeShan, 1982). They claim a place for reductionism within holistic health as a method of study, but not as a mode of therapy.

Generally, holists like to avoid that which requires dissection and analysis. When this is unavoidable, an attempt is made to indicate how attention to the part contributes to the well-being of the whole. For example, in the case of a patient suffering from bacterial pneumonia, standard antibiotic therapy would be considered appropriate. But the holistic practitioner would also view this interaction with the client as an opportunity to explore concerns about environmental hazards (air pollution), personal health habits (smoking), and coping mechanisms (response to stress).

2. *"MIND" AND "BODY" ARE ARTIFICIAL DISTINCTIONS THAT INTERFERE WITH OUR UNDERSTANDING OF MAN'S ESSENTIAL INTEGRITY.* When attempting to explain how this notion (which to them is clearly a truism) has somehow escaped the notice of the medical community, holists always hark back to Descartes. They suggest that the physiological bias of Western medicine originated with Cartesian dualism and has ever since had a pernicious effect on the quality of health care. Medical doctors now care for our bodies, and psychiatrists treat disorders of the mind. However, because the duality does not exist in nature, but is only imagined, the person is not necessarily healed when the part is attended to.

This statement goes beyond asserting that man is more than the sum of his parts to claim that in fact he has no parts. Some authors have tried to indicate this by using such terms as mind/body system (Capra, 1982). Others discuss man's body, mind, and spirit, but emphasize that these are but aspects of a unified being. It is believed that our understanding is distorted by our limited vocabulary, which fails to provide us with terms denoting wholeness.

Health

1. *GOOD HEALTH IS MORE THAN PHYSICAL
WELL-BEING. IT IS A FUNCTION OF BALANCE AMONG
THE PHYSICAL, MENTAL, AND SPIRITUAL ASPECTS
OF A PERSON IN HARMONY WITH THE ENVIRON-
MENT.* Nearly every definition of holistic health includes
a statement to this effect. Its intent is to enlarge the standard definition of health as a satisfactory physical condition to include all aspects of being. Bodily functioning
alone is not considered an adequate indicator of health.
It is but one factor in the body-mind-spirit complex that
must be maintained in a dynamic balance. Dysfunction
in one system inevitably leads to a deterioration of the
health of the organism as a whole.

This use of terms denoting parts is an example of the
problematic nature of the previous dictum that mind and
body are artificial distinctions without true human coun-
terparts. It is often suggested that, though a person may
have aspects or functions reflected by these terms, they
are so complexly related as to be virtually indistinguishable, and cannot be isolated for analysis without violating
the integrity of the whole. Land (1980) states that "a major theme in the holistic health movement is the integration of body, mind and spirit. Each functions with the
other as a whole system that is not reducible to the sum
of its parts. A major goal in our new awareness is to
begin to understand the nature of these interrelation-
ships" (p. 135).

Health of the body, though important to holists, is felt
to have received undue, even exclusive, attention from
conventional health-care practitioners. Holists have
therefore focused on what is variously termed the mental, emotional, or psychological aspect of illness. A consensus exists that all illness has a psychological

component, but disagreement exists over the importance of its influence. Flynn (1980) claims that "each condition of illness or health has a greater or lesser psychosocial or physiological component to begin with, and in the course of every condition there is interaction between the two" (p. 37). She conceptualizes the etiologies of illness as occurring on a continuum ranging from purely organic to purely psychosocial.

Others believe that psychological factors play a significant, if not primary, role in all illness. Capra (1982) represents this view:

> When the systems view of mind is adopted, it becomes obvious that any illness has mental aspects. Getting sick and healing are both integral parts of an organism's self-organization, and since mind represents the dynamics of this self-organization, the processes of getting sick and of healing are essentially mental phenomena. Because mentation is a multileveled pattern of processes, most of them taking place in the unconscious realm, we are not always fully aware of how we move in and out of illness, but this not alter the fact that illness is a mental phenomenon in its very essence. (p. 327)

The spirit, the component of the health triad usually mentioned last, is given less attention than body and mind. Although they assert its importance, holists have little to say about how spiritual breakdown manifests itself as a health problem and how it can be treated. Perhaps this is a result of the failure to define the spirit itself adequately. Land (1980) notes that "there are many notions about what constitutes the spirit. . . . The concept of spirit may . . . include consciousness, environmental sensitivity, and a sense of connectedness to all parts of the universe. Many thinkers have equated total consciousness or enlightenment with total integration, harmony, or balance of body, mind and spirit" (pp. 135–136). The concept of spirit is nebulous in the holistic literature and, though it is nearly always cited as important to health, it is seldom discussed at length, or else is included in the consideration of psychological aspects.

Finally, holists point out that even people who are functioning well mentally, physically, and spiritually cannot be healthy unless they are interacting appropriately with the environment. It must provide them with certain necessities, and they in turn must not abuse it. Environment is defined broadly and may include other persons as well as natural surroundings. It most often is considered to extend beyond the individual's immediate locale and may be inclusive of the cosmos.

2. *HEALTH HAS POSITIVE ATTRIBUTES AND IS NOT SIMPLY THE ABSENCE OF DISEASE*. From the holistic perspective, failure to identify pathology in any of the areas mentioned above does not constitute sufficient evidence that the subjects are healthy. They may be free of all organic and psychological disease, and still not have achieved a state of health. Healthy persons have energy and optimism, are goal-directed, and are engaged in fulfilling their own potentials. They have much in common with Maslow's self-actualizer.

Because health is commonly identified as the lack of disease, many people accept their mediocre conditions and fail to engage in those activities that could help them to achieve true health. The holists believe that conventional health-care practitioners contribute to this misunderstanding by limiting their practices to the treatment of objective signs of disease. These practitioners view other kinds of complaints with disdain and relegate them to the care of the clergy, psychiatrists, and social workers, thereby widening the Cartesian split even further.

Holists would like to see as much attention given to health promotion as is presently given to the elimination of symptoms.

3. *ILL-HEALTH, OR DISEASE, IS MULTICAUSAL AND CANNOT BE ASSIGNED A SINGLE ETIOLOGY.* Disease causation is not regarded as a matter of simple cause and effect. This is the model used in conventional Western medicine. It assumes that every disease has an identifiable cause, and probably a single cure as well. Germ theory is based on this model and has been enormously successful in contributing to the control of infectious disease. But holists note that not all diseases are appropriate to this model. LeShan (1982), for example, points out that research has failed to yield a single cause for any of the degenerative diseases.

The claim of multicausality is closely related to the notion of man as a mind-body-spirit complex. According to holistic thought, each aspect is likely to be involved in an illness. It is the interaction between the agent and the person that is responsible for the development of illness. Lappé (1979) states: "In the holistic view, disease processes should be understood in a broader context than linear causation; that is, as resulting from the interactions of multiple factors. . . . Many diseases previously thought to be caused solely by outside agents actually result from a combination of internal *and* external factors" (pp. 475 and 476). An example commonly given to illustrate the limitations of single-agent theory is the situation in which a number of people have been exposed to a particular bacteria, but only a few contract an infection. Holists insist that other variables besides the infectious organism determine which persons will succumb to the disease.

As Mattson (1982) has noted, stress theory, as formulated by Hans Selye, is used by holists to explain the nature of these variables. According to Selye (1976), any stimulus to which a person is subjected is capable of contributing to disease if the individual's response is maladaptive. Thus, both physical and mental stimuli, regardless of whether they are considered as desirable or to be avoided, are potentially disease-producing.

4. *BECAUSE ILLNESS SIGNALS AN IMBALANCE, IT CAN BE A LEARNING EXPERIENCE, PROVIDING PEOPLE WITH AN OPPORTUNITY TO ALTER HARMFUL BEHAVIORS.* When the delicate balance of body-mind-spirit is disturbed, the resulting disease is a warning. Persons who attend to it may be able to regain their health by making adjustments in their habits. Thus, disease is not viewed as entirely negative.

Some holists believe that the manifestations of illness have symbolic significance. M. Ferguson (1980) claims that "we may make our metaphors literal" by developing acne when we feel "picked on" or experiencing somatic versions of a broken heart or a pain in the neck (p. 253).

The more widely held view is that, though symptoms are not always symbolically organ-specific, they do reflect problems that are potentially treatable by individuals themselves through alterations in life-style. Illness is therefore characterized as an opportunity for change, growth, and learning. The role of the health-care provider is that of an educator who can help clients recognize how their behaviors have contributed to the development of disease and who then assists them in learning new patterns of behavior that will enable them to restore the balance necessary for good health. Gordon (1981) says that holistic practitioners help patients see the relationship between psychosocial stresses and illness and use the event of illness to motivate their clients to reevaluate attitudes and behaviors.

The goal of this type of education is not simply to return patients to their pre-illness conditions, but to allow them to achieve a state of ever greater well-being. It is hoped that they will use the experience not only to recognize and gain control over destructive habits, but to gain insight into the values they hold and the relationships that are significant in their lives (Flynn, 1980).

Health Care

1. *THE PREVENTION OF ILLNESS AND THE MAINTENANCE OF HEALTH ARE MORE IMPORTANT THAN THE TREATMENT OF DISEASE.* Just as health is considered to be more than the absence of disease within the holistic framework, so is health care considered to involve more than the treatment of disease. The traditional methods of conventional medicine are regarded as inadequate to the task of improving the health of the population. LaLonde (1980), in his study of Canadian health care, suggests that further improvements in the health of the citizens will not be attained through the use of biomedical interventions but through a decrease in self-imposed risks, betterment of the environment, and an improved understanding of the nature of human health.

Holists would like to see health care as a praxis rather than a service. Health itself is not seen as a passive state but as a condition to be achieved and maintained. Although holistic practitioners may treat illness, they prefer to concentrate on preventing its occurrence, which may be regarded as a failure on the part of either client or practitioner. (This would seem to contradict the notion of illness as opportunity.) Twemlow (1981) says that a "global approach to holistic health will have to address two issues: (1) how to stop people from doing things that are detrimental to their health; and (2) how to engage people in alternative behaviors that will increase their health and well being" (p. 450). Trying to treat illness after it has occurred may be seen as akin to shutting the barn door after the cows have escaped.

2. *TO BE EFFECTIVE, HEALTH CARE MUST FOCUS ON THE WHOLE PERSON, NOT JUST THE DISEASED PART.* This is another statement rejecting reductionism. People are wholes and must be treated in their entirety. Medical care that treats symptoms and diseases is unacceptable if social and psychological factors are ignored because the overt manifestations of disease are but the tip of the larger pathological iceberg. Capra (1982) states:

> Not everything that alleviates suffering temporarily is necessarily good. If the intervention is carried out without taking other aspects of the illness into account, the result will generally be unhealthy for the patient in the long run. . . . Surgical treatment of a blocked artery may temporarily alleviate pain but will not make the person well. The surgical intervention merely treats a local effect of a systemic disorder that will continue until the underlying problems are identified and resolved. (p. 157)

To illustrate this point, holists frequently employ a simile in which the client is likened to a broken automobile or other machine, and the practitioner is compared to a repairman or mechanic whose task it is to "fix" the broken part. It is suggested that people, unlike automobiles, require more sophisticated forms of healing than is indicated by the "repair" model.

3. *INDIVIDUALS ARE LARGELY RESPONSIBLE FOR MAINTAINING THEIR OWN HEALTH.* This is one of the most fiercely held tenets of the movement and is related

to several of the previous statements. It is an extension of the assumption that every illness has multiple causes, at least some of which are under the control of the individual. Psychological factors are regarded as particularly important and are believed to be frequently overlooked. Ill people are supposed to be able to alter the course of their diseases by psychic maneuvers. A positive attitude is essential and may be supplemented by such techniques as hypnosis, relaxation, or meditation.

Physical factors are also felt to be significant to good health. Individuals are held responsible for eating a balanced diet, obtaining adequate rest and exercise, and avoiding harmful substances such as tobacco and excessive alcohol. They are also held accountable if they choose to expose themselves to unnecessary hazards, for example by not wearing automobile seat belts.

Personal responsibility for health also ties in with the notion that illness may be an opportunity for learning. P. Albright (1980b) states that "self-development toward the goals of individual responsibility and vibrant health is . . . an educational process in which people learn to tune in to various signals and to adjust their lives accordingly" (p. 36).

Opinion is divided regarding how far personal responsibility extends. Few go so far as to suggest that people have absolute control over their well-being. Many writers are careful to point out that some influences, such as air pollution, may be beyond the control of the individual.

4. *ALTHOUGH CONVENTIONAL MEDICAL CARE IS USEFUL, AND SOMETIMES NECESSARY, SELF-CARE IS PREFERABLE IN MANY INSTANCES.* Self-responsibility involves not only taking measures to prevent illness, but also engaging in therapeutic procedures for the

treatment of disease. The authority to cure, once restricted to physicians, has devolved on the patient.

In general, holists are suspicious, if not outright rejecting, of Western medicine (also known as conventional, orthodox, cosmopolitan, traditional, or biomedicine). They seek to wrest control of health care from medical experts and offer it instead to patients, or clients. T. Ferguson (1980) says: "Holistic health proposes that our health system needs a new map. Self-care suggests that the wrong person has been holding the map" (p. 393).

Persons are encouraged to learn as much as possible about providing their own health care. Medical practitioners are to be consulted as teachers and colleagues. There is, however, general agreement that the contributions of Western medicine are significant and ought not to be abandoned. Physicians in the movement, in particular, are eager to point out that holistic and conventional medicine are not mutually exclusive, but may complement one another (Sobel, 1979).

Nevertheless, doctors are urged to relinquish the role of authoritarian experts and to work with patients on a more collegial basis. It is assumed that patients are the true experts because they have direct access to the subjective data of their bodies and minds. Only when serious illness or trauma occurs are physicians to assume the role of expert technicians. As one holistic enthusiast said, "If I fall off my motorcycle and break my leg, don't take me to the health food store! I want to go to the nearest hospital emergency room" (Albright, P., 1980a, p. 265).

5. *THE HEALTH-CARE PRACTITIONER IS NOT SIMPLY AN EXPERT OR TECHNICIAN, BUT IS AN AGENT WHO HELPS ILL PERSONS MOBILIZE THEIR OWN HEALING POWERS.* Healing comes from within. All persons have the ability to use their own resources to foster

health and fight disease. Holistic practitioners believe that their own efforts are but the mediate cause of recovery. Their job is to teach or facilitate the patients' use of their innate healing abilities. Frequent reference is made in the literature to the Hippocratic concept of *vis medicatrix naturae*—the healing power of nature.

Faith healing, in which cure is effected without any physical or pharmacological intervention, offers a particularly clear example of how a practitioner may attempt to stimulate a restorative response from the patient. According to Dubos, "Faith healing in any form always depends on self-healing" (1979b, p. x). Disagreement prevails about whether the ability to promote healing is a special gift or is a quality that can be acquired by anyone.

More direct interventions such as acupuncture, massage, and dietary changes, or even surgery and drugs, may be helpful in restoring well-being. Nevertheless, these techniques are merely aids to the natural healing ability inherent in each of us.

6. *CARING IS A SIGNIFICANT COMPONENT OF THE HEALING PROCESS.* The healing just discussed cannot be effected through any particular therapy unless its use is accompanied by a caring attitude on the part of the healer. Holistic practitioners endeavor to establish a relationship with their clients based on genuine concern, warmth, even love. Conventional medicine is criticized for its emphasis on maintaining a neutral, "scientific" stance toward clients as represented by the standard admonition not to "get involved" with patients. Even therapists who maintain a respectful and cordial relationship with their clients cannot expect to be effective if they are at the same time detached from clients' subjective experiences. The best holistic techniques will fail in the hands of an uncaring practitioner. Solomon

(1980) goes so far as to claim that love (which he calls the X-factor) is a requisite for healing:

> Regardless of your practice, your specialty, or your technique, there is a common factor in healing, the single most important factor. It is, in fact, the *one* that makes healing work. . . . If this X-factor is not present, you won't heal no matter how well you have mastered your techniques. But, if you do have the X-factor, you probably will heal in spite of your techniques. (p. 14)

Holistic practitioners may spend a great deal of time exploring their own personalities, value systems, and emotional responses to clients in order to become more able to experience and express caring feelings towards those who seek them out for treatment.

7. *UNORTHODOX DIAGNOSTIC TECHNIQUES AND THERAPIES THAT ELICIT A POSITIVE RESPONSE FROM THE PATIENT MAY BE LEGITIMATE, EVEN IF THEIR EFFICACY HAS NOT BEEN CONFIRMED BY SCIENTIFIC TESTING. LOW-TECHNOLOGY, NON INVASIVE, "NATURAL" REMEDIES ARE ESPECIALLY DESIRABLE.* The term "holistic medicine" frequently evokes among the lay population images of eccentric and untrained therapists practicing exotic remedies. It is true that those in the movement have evinced much interest in "alternative" (non-Western) modes of diagnosis and treatment. Some techniques such as iridology—the diagnosis of disease by examination of the iris—are considered bizarre even by many self-proclaimed holists. Other, like acupuncture, are gradually being admitted into mainstream medicine.

A hallmark of holism is an openness to anything that "works," even if the mechanism is unclear. Canton

(1980) exhorts physicians to be tolerant of new practices in the hope that they might prove helpful:

> The human body and mind are extremely complex. The patient has a right to try other modalities. Most of the time, it is not a matter of life or death. Open-mindedness may mean making a referral, or waiting while the patient explores other modalities, or learning a technique such as acupuncture, hypnosis, biofeedback, or dream interpretation. (p. 172)

Scientific validation of efficacy may be sought in order to establish credibility with the public or the conventional medical community, but is not considered a prerequisite to use. It is felt that not all therapeutic results are easily quantified. Patients' statements that they feel better may be regarded as sufficient evidence that procedures are effective. Pelletier (1979a) contends that "caution needs to be exercised in evaluating any clinical procedure, but it is equally important not to discard positive clinical outcome because it does not appear compatible with the prevailing scientific paradigm" (p. 15).

Holists point out that not all conventional therapies are well understood. The mechanism by which aspirin relieves pain, for example, remains a mystery. Nor are all of scientific medicine's remedies safe; iatrogenic (treatment-induced) complications abound, and sometimes the consequences of treatment are worse than the disease itself. Holistic practitioners try to obey the injunction to "do no harm" by using what they believe to be low-risk procedures. Many of these derive from traditional healing systems and folk medicine. They are often described as "natural." This term has not been well defined. It may refer to a remedy used by primitive peoples, to a substance found occurring in nature, or simply to a procedure that does not involve machines or drugs.

Many holistic practitioners seek to include all effective forms of therapy in their practice. Use of only conventional or only alternative methods is seen as unnecessarily limiting. Nevertheless, a distinct bias is evident within the movement against the highly technological interventions of Western medicine.

Summary

Among the uninitiated, a frequent response to the mention of the holistic health movement is to acknowledge familiarity with the term, but express uncertainty as to what it denotes: "Just what *is* holistic health, anyway?" In spite of the loose association among advocates of holistic health, I think it is fair to state that they and their efforts constitute a movement, for which the tenets just discussed provide some coherence. Although there is diversity in current holistic thought, common themes do emerge; shared assumptions develop.

Attempts have been made to define holistic health and the movement it has generated. Most have appeared in a paragraph or even a single sentence proclaiming unity of body, mind, and spirit. Others have gone further and have listed beliefs regarded as central. A few have suggested that holistic health is difficult to describe, let alone define, because it is only a "perspective" or "orientation." Thus far, none of these answers has been satisfactory. At best, they are unfocused and incomplete. This may be considered excusable and even to be expected in a movement so young, one that is still evolving. But the authors seem prematurely satisfied with their

efforts. This is partly the result of the element of evan-
gelism associated with the movement: one doesn't prove
or explain, one believes.

The failure to articulate basic concepts must be viewed
as unacceptable in a movement that lays claim to us body
and soul. Nevertheless, we are drawn to it by the promises it makes. The present health-care system is indeed
overpriced, impersonal, and often ineffective. We turn
like plants to the sun toward a system that pledges to
unify this fragmented arrangement. In our desire for the
rewards offered, we may neglect to examine the premises
on which they are based.

As holists themselves so often point out, it is the movement's philosophy that dictates its practices. Therefore,
we must first understand its thinking if we are to fairly
evaluate it. And it must be evaluated on its own terms.
Because of the dearth of serious discussion in the holistic
literature, this means we are forced to rely on the slogans
it uses in lieu of solid argument. It is, perhaps, the apparent *reasonableness* of the statements that has allowed
them to escape any genuinely critical analysis. There
seems to be a commonsensical truth to them that is difficult to deny. Who is willing to claim that illness is a
purely physical phenomenon or that the prevention of
illness is unimportant? Is it possible to make a case
against the belief in personal responsibility for health?
The holistic slogans appear to be almost self-evidently
true.

For the doubters, the holists are able to supply numerous examples in support of their claims. Does not
everyone agree, for instance, that people can ruin their
health with bad habits? Indeed, don't we each know
someone who has done so? Of course, one of the criticisms lodged against the movement has been that its
"evidence" is largely anecdotal. This criticism may be

justified regarding particular therapies that have not been subjected to scientific testing.

Many of the tenets, however, do not lend themselves to testing, but would best be supported by argument. The holists have not offered more than superficial support for their tenets. A statement such as "The prevention of disease is more important than cure" is felt to be a simple truth, easily understood and not requiring any explanation or analysis. On the surface, it is difficult to contradict. Sensitive practitioners recognize that preventing illness is to be desired over waiting until it occurs, then treating it. Still, little thought may be given to what the full significance of this statement may be. Such is the power of this kind of slogan that to oppose it is to expose oneself as either ignorant or uncaring. Most of these statements contain a germ of truth, and it is often enough to carry their entire import.

The remaining chapters in this book will assess both the accuracy and the utility of these statements as they are used by holists and will consider the possibility that some of them have already become slogans of the type Scheffler describes. A number have already found their way into popular usage; some are becoming accepted by the conventional medical community. A few have already achieved the status of truisms, and those who use them may be unaware of their origins as holistic formulations. All of this is taking place without serious examination. Can these statements provide a sound basis for practice? What are the possible consequences of adopting them for individuals, for society, and for the health-care professions? These questions will be considered next.

3

Health and Illness

Health. Americans today spend increasing amounts of
time thinking, talking, reading, and writing about it. We
spend considerable energy worrying about it and trying
to protect it by various means. And we spend enormous
amounts of money trying to restore it when it deterio-
rates. For some, health represents the highest value, the
most precious commodity; it is virtually the sine qua non
of a profitable human life.

Our concern for our health has developed a rather desperate quality. We must preserve it above all else and at
any cost. We are increasingly beset by anxieties regarding
the possibility of becoming ill. No longer do we take
health for granted until illness occurs. Now we are alert
to the slightest change in our well-being, terrified that
we may find some deviation from the norm.

Anxiously, health-conscious citizens monitor their
pulses, nutritional intakes, bowel patterns, sleep habits,
exercise levels, social lives, and sexual activities. Nothing
escapes their notice. But they do not stop at assessing
health status. They actively seek to maintain health by
engaging in a stupefying variety of "health-promoting"
behavior. They jog, practice transcendental meditation,
and do not smoke or drink. They eat a carefully balanced

diet that is supplemented with a personal pharmacopoeia of tablets and powders. Finally, they rely on health practitioners to provide them with checkups and screenings that will eliminate the possibility they have overlooked some disorder lurking in their bodies, waiting to rob them of health.

Yet, despite all the effort they put into protecting their health, these people remain uneasy. They can never be certain of remaining well. Further, they are nagged by the suspicion that, though they are well, they could be better. Perhaps it is not enough to be simply free from disease; perhaps they ought to be striving for an even stronger body, a sharper mind, and more satisfying human relationships. Thus, what in another time was considered the blessing or gift of good health has become the never-ending struggle for good health. How is it that we have become so grim in our pursuit of well-being? This chapter will seek to demonstrate that our concern with personal health is largely a by-product of the holistic health movement.

Changing Concepts of Health and Illness

To a child, people are healthy when they "feel good" and sick when they "catch" something. The distinction between health and disease is not always so clear. Health is defined differently by different groups, in different times, and from different perspectives. Even individuals have personal definitions that may not be consonant with the prevailing one.

What is illness to one person may be an annoyance to another, and considered normal by a third. So it is with societies as well. Dubos (1959) points out that "modern man looks with dismay on the fact that syphilis, malaria, yaws, intestinal disorders, etc., are so common in some areas of the world as not to be regarded as diseases. Yet he accepts as part and parcel of a normal life baldness, poor eyesight, chronic sinusitis, and other bodily defects which might be regarded as handicaps or even as repulsive traits in other cultural contexts" (p. 218).

Ideas regarding disease causation, too, have changed over time. Ancient peoples were likely to assign supernatural causes to disease, and many of today's diagnosticians use the scientific method to determine the etiologies of illness. Even during the same historical period, many theories of disease causation coexist. Anthropologist George Murdock (1980) has listed thirteen categories of theories extant: infection, stress, organic deterioration, accident, overt human aggression, fate, ominous sensations, contagion, mystical retribution, soul loss, spirit aggression, sorcery, and witchcraft.

Occasionally, proponents of opposing theories collide. Betz (1978) describes the results of such a collision between university researchers and American Indians in the southwestern United States. The researchers were interested in investigating Chagas' disease among the Indian population. The paradigm of Western medicine embraced by the researchers indicated that this disease, which causes cardiac disorders and sometimes death, is attributable to the parasite *T. cruzi*. The Indians, however, believed the cause was disturbing the power residing in such things as animals, plants, crystal rocks, thunder, and lightning. The researchers found the Indians resentful of their investigations, partly because of the fundamental differences in perceptions of disease causation.

Another example of the difficulty in reconciling perceptions that are at variance with one another is the confusion that can result when Latin American patients who subscribe to the humoral concept present themselves for conventional medical treatment. This concept classifies both symptoms and treatments as either hot or cold, a hot treatment being appropriate to a cold symptom and vice versa. Thus, a Puerto Rican client may reject a hot treatment (penicillin) to treat a disease accompanied by fever (Logan, 1978). Similarly, Brandt (1978) noted that Navajo patients being cared for by non-Navajo health-care workers may withdraw from treatment if the cause of the health problem is described primarily in terms of pathophysiology because the Navajo believe that disease is caused by disharmony among emotions, body, spirit, and nature.

Even within a given culture, however, notions of health and disease may appear radically different when viewed from selected perspectives. Hence, the sociologist looks at people's ability to perform roles and tasks (Talcott Parsons), the psychologist determines the extent to which their needs are being met (Abraham Maslow), the theologian examines their relationships to God (Martin Buber), and the physician scrutinizes their bodies for evidence of mechanical failure.

It is not unusual to find an individual who maintains a number of perspectives concurrently. A woman who holds a predominantly religious world view, for example, may find a means of reconciling other perspectives under the umbrella of "God's will." Therefore, although she subscribes to the germ theory, she will interpret her ear infection as an event ordained by God. Similarly, she may seek the services of a psychiatric social worker for her unwed, pregnant daughter in the belief that God wishes her to use every possible resource to protect her family's welfare.

It is becoming much less common to find people willing to assign disease causation to a single agent—God did it, a germ did it, the evil eye did it. Multiple causation theories are dominant. They propose that "illness rarely, if ever, results from a single, discrete, disease-causing agent acting upon an otherwise normal and healthy person. Instead, multiple-causation theories postulate that human beings exist in and respond to external physical and social environments" (Sakalys, 1981, p. 5).

Neither are definitions of health as simple as they once were. At one time, they closely approximated the child's definition of "not sick." Such an approach is now considered unacceptably narrow by most health-care practitioners. Typically, they argue for expanding the definition on the grounds that the absence of disease does not guarantee that a person is exercising his or her full human potential for a satisfying life. Health, they claim, has positive attributes that make it more than the lack of something else. Further, it is felt to be multifaceted and not merely a reflection of physical well-being. The World Health Organization (WHO) offered such a definition when it described health as a state of "complete physical, mental, and social well-being, and not merely the absence of disease and infirmity" (1947).

This definition is so global that one suspects that few persons can qualify as well. Mechanic (1978) protests:

> The broadness of this definition makes it inapplicable for differentiating the healthy from the sick in an operational sense, and thus it is not very useful except as a guide to the broad dimensions of health and a reminder that even physical well-being is dependent on the contexts in

which we live, our associations with others, and the
physical and social assaults to which our living situation
exposes us. (p. 53)

Although the WHO definition has been widely criticized
as vague and even "dangerous" (Callahan, 1977), its influence has been enormous. It is widely quoted in the
health-care literature and has filtered down to the lay
population as well. This group, though perhaps unfa-
miliar with the text, has widely accepted its basic premise: health involves the "whole" person, not just the
body.

The Holistic View

The appeal of the WHO definition to holistic health
advocates is obvious. The rallying cry "Health is more
than the absence of disease!" rings throughout the literature. Most holistic definitions of health include these
or similar words. One version holds that wellness is a
"state of mental, physical, and social well-being, not just
the absence of disease. It is more than being well; it is
having the energy and enthusiasm for life's activities"
(in Ardell, 1978, p. 5). Often an attempt is made to identify the positive aspects of health that differentiate it from
illness. Brallier (1978) offers the following:

Holistic health is an ongoing sense of finely tuned wellness, which involves not only excellent care of the physical body but also care of ourselves in such a way that we
nurture our capacity to be mentally alert and creative as
well as emotionally stable and satisfied. It involves the
feeling of wholeness we can gain from having defined
our philosophy of life and purpose in life. (p. 645)

Definitions such as these have been criticized (like the WHO version from which they are derived) as being too broad and too vague. Because they believe health is complex, holists try to include in their descriptions the many aspects of which it is comprised. The results are elaborate definitions that may vary in scope from author to author. That health is more than the absence of disease is accepted as a given; less agreement exists on which positive factors accrue to health.

As Engelhardt (1981) notes regarding the WHO statement, global statements about health are so idealistic that they exclude most people from being considered healthy. Nevertheless, they serve the purpose of calling attention to nonphysical health influences. Certainly the evidence is overwhelming that social, psychological, and environmental events can contribute to overt physical illness. This has long been accepted by epidemiologists, who evaluate the etiologies of disease in terms of agent, host, and environment (Leavell, 1958). Furthermore, it is clear that the subjective experience of illness can occur in the absence of identifiable pathology. Conversely, a person with clinical evidence of disease may have a sense of being well (Engel, G., 1980). In questioning the adequacy of holistic conceptions of health, I am not denying the influence of nonphysical factors on health. To suggest, however, that those factors are the same as health may be an error.

Concepts should serve to order our thinking. Much debate has occurred over whether health is best conceived as a scientific concept that has precise parameters, or a social concept whose meaning is determined by groups. Both understandings may be useful. Scientific concepts serve to direct our investigations, and social concepts help us to explain behavior as well as to make decisions. The holistic concept does neither. It might be described as an idiosyncratic concept, that is, one that is understood only as it applies to an individual. In Braillier's terms, for example, health involves a sense of satisfaction and a feeling of wholeness, both subjective phenomena that are entirely unique to each person and unavailable to an outside observer. Thus, the holistic understanding of health is idiosyncratic, relative, and not useful as a concept.

In trying to formulate a concept that is less global and less personal, yet which accounts for extra-physical factors, it may be necessary to distinguish between health and well-being. The two are necessarily associated (recall the child's understanding of health with "feeling good"), but may not be one and the same. The holists are correct in assuming a relationship and in insisting that subjective data receive a fair hearing. It is often pain, malaise, or psychic distress that alerts us to incipient illness. Conventional medicine, too, recognizes the importance of "symptoms" (subjective manifestations of disease) as well as "signs" (objective manifestations).

But, although a sense of well-being may be an indicator of health, it is not the same as health. Kopelman and Moskop (1981) ask:

> If health means well-being, then is anyone who does anything that makes us feel better or instructs us in activities that would do so (sailing, skiing), engaging in healing practices? . . . One cannot doubt that sometimes music, dance and recreational sports contribute more to our well-being than going to a clinic. Is that which makes one feel better or promotes well-being . . . to qualify as a health practice? (p. 223)

Many holists would answer these questions in the affirmative because they consider well-being and health to be inextricably bound up in one another; if one does not feel well, then by definition one is not healthy. It would be more helpful to consider health and well-being to be related but distinct phenomena, each of which is affected by similar variables.

For example, it has been demonstrated that severe social stressors are associated with the onset of disease (Holmes and Rahe, 1967). These same stressors can also lead to feelings of unhappiness. A problem arises when a single stressor is believed to have consequences for only a single area of human functioning. That is, if I have a high-pressure job, I may experience an exacerbation of my diabetic condition (disruption of health) or experience feelings of tension and anxiety (disruption of well-being), or both. True, those unhappy feelings may themselves impinge on my health, and this is the cause of much confusion. It is difficult to sort out the cause and effect in many situations, but holists only confuse the issue further by insisting that everything which impinges on well-being is impinging on health as well.

Definitions of health and illness have been proposed, questioned, reformulated, and generally struggled with by conventional providers as well as by holists. Contrary to what some holists have suggested, many are unwilling to define health as the lack of physical problems. But to frame the definition of health in negative terms—to say that it is *not* just the absence of disease—is not to say what health *is*, and this is the subject of much debate.

Besson (1967) describes six situations in which the health status of an individual is ambiguous:

1. The well patient with subclinical disease.
2. The well patient who is exposed to risk, such as smoking, and may therefore be in the incubation stage of disease.

3. The well patient who is temporarily overwhelmed by life's problems.
4. The well patient who prefers the sick role.
5. The sick patient who refuses the sick role.
6. The patient who cannot be evaluated because he never presents for treatment (p. 1902).

According to some holistic formulations, each of these persons would be regarded as ill.

But is illness the same as disease? Eisenberg (1977) makes an interesting distinction: "Patients suffer 'illnesses'; physicians diagnose and treat 'diseases'. . . . Illnesses are *experiences* of disvalued changes in states of being and in social function; diseases, in the scientific paradigm of modern medicine, are *abnormalities* in the *structure* and *function* of body organs and systems" (p. 11).

Given this distinction, some conventional providers would equate health with the absence of disease (Callahan, 1973), but others would insist that health requires the absence of *both* disease and illness. The latter view is closest to the holistic view, particularly when the "disvalued changes in states of being" that constitute illness are not only the result of physical disease, but also of other life experiences, such as an unhappy marriage. J. A. Smith (1981) labels this broad concept of health the "eudaimonistic" model, and asserts that those using it equate health with "general well being and self-realization" (p. 44). The eudaimonistic model is often used by conventional providers, but the parallels with holistic definitions are obvious.

It bears repeating that many of the ideas claimed by holists have a history that pre-dates the modern holistic health movement. Contemporary conventional providers subscribe to many of them. However, when one of these slogans ("Health is more than the absence of disease") appears in the conventional literature, it may be difficult to determine whether the writer is aware of the history of the idea within the tradition of his discipline, or whether he or she is responding to the influence of the modern holists. Regardless, however, of whether one refers to eudaimonistic or to holistic health, the concept is too broad to be useful.

Health may indeed be more than the absence of disease, but how much more? More in what ways? And what human phenomena are to be excluded from the concept? The holists have made a contribution by framing it in more than physical terms, but health cannot be the "whole of everything" to recall James's words. If their concept is to be taken seriously, they will have to fit it with some limits. Their presently unwieldy, all-inclusive concept has already created some difficulties.

The Creation of New Health Needs

The enlarged concept of health regards all aspects of a person's being as part of his or her health, and requires that all parts be scrutinized, adjusted, and set in balance with one another. Health is unattainable in the face of unresolved family problems, a sedentary life-style, or oppressive social conditions. Only when "All's right with the world" can a person's health flourish. And it must flourish, not simply be adequate. Lack of symptoms is not considered a significant indicator of the vibrant well-being that is sought. R. C. Fox (1977) says that "increasingly, health has become a coded way of referring to an individually, socially, or cosmically ideal state of affairs" (p. 15).

No longer are a "sensible" life-style and medical attention for acute illnesses considered sufficient to protect health. As the definition of health has expanded, so too have the requisite number of "health behaviors." Individuals are forced to spend even greater amounts of time and energy attending to their health in order to have a sense of well-being and freedom from anxiety. Crawford (1980) refers to this as "healthism," which he defines as "the preoccupation with personal health as a primary—often *the* primary—focus for the definition and achievement of well-being" (p. 368).

Holists believe that if they attend carefully enough to their "whole" selves, they will be healthy. No part, however small, can be ignored. They consider illness a reflection of neglect or failure to meet one of their many needs. It is a mistaken belief. Man has never been autonomous to the point that he is free from the unpredictable forces of nature. He is perhaps subject as well to the whims of fate and the will of God. No matter how carefully we engineer our lives, illness and death remain part of them. Dubos (1959) claims that the dream that man can achieve a state of perfect health and happiness can never be realized:

> Life is an adventure in a world where nothing is static; where unpredictable and ill-understood events constitute dangers that must be overcome, often blindly and at great cost. . . . The more creative the individual the less he can hope to avoid danger. . . . Complete and lasting freedom from disease is but a dream remembered from imaginings of a Garden of Eden designed for the welfare of man. (pp. 1–2)

The holists, however, are undeterred. They persist in their attempts to reconstruct the Garden of Eden. But they seek not merely freedom from physical disease. It is not enough that they have food, clothing, and shelter. They must also have entertainment, intellectual stimulation, social intercourse, spiritual enrichment, and a congenial environment. These are no longer considered part of the "good life," but are indispensable to the healthy life.

These desires are not unique to the holist, of course. As Dubos points out, "It is a universal trait among men that as soon as their physiological needs are satisfied, they develop new wishes and urges, which in turn are soon replaced by other desires" (p. 53). What is peculiar to holists is their proclivity for transforming "wants" into "needs." This is a direct outcome of their global conception of health. People who see health as absence of disease have fewer health needs. Holists, who see everything that impinges upon them as affecting their health, have to satisfy many more needs in order to meet their multiple criteria for health. Thus, some individuals may feel well if they are not actively ill and their physiological needs are adequately met, but others may not consider themselves healthy if they cannot express themselves creatively. Illich (1977b) says, "When I learned to speak . . . 'need' was mainly used as a verb. The expressions 'I have a problem' or 'I have a need' both sounded silly. . . . During the second half of my life, to be 'needy' became respectable. . . . To be ignorant or unconvinced of one's own needs has become the unforgiveable antisocial act" (pp. 30 and 31).

Holists are unlikely to be ignorant of their health needs, though this requires greater vigilance all the time, as those needs keep multiplying. Unable to handle them all themselves, they turn for help to experts who materialize with each new need. "New pundits constantly jump on the bandwagon of the therapeutic-care provider:

educators, social workers, the military, town-planners, judges, policemen, and their ilk have obviously made it" (Illich, 1977b, p. 26). These professionals assist their clients to recognize that what they have been considering as either desires or difficulties are actually needs. The assertiveness training instructor, for example, can reinterpret his clients' desire to be in control when interacting with their bosses as a "healthy need for mastery."

Unhappiness, anxiety, and difficulties need no longer be attributed to personal failure, God's will, or simply the human condition. Rather, they may be considered as a symptom of unmet needs. We justify even our crassest desires as needs. The father who enjoys the status earned by sending his child to an exclusive private school may justify it on the basis of the child's intellectual needs. Rieff (1968) believes that, "difficult as the modern cultural condition may be, I doubt that Western men can be persuaded again to the Greek opinion that the secret of happiness is to have as few needs as possible" (p. 17). Indeed, our perceived needs continue to proliferate.

The Expansion of the Sick Role

As wants are transmogrified into needs, discomfort becomes disease. As the definition of health expands, fewer people are able to feel healthy. The holistic health movement, which purports to help individuals become well, instead is responsible for increasing the amount of illness experienced by its adherents. Because the standards of the holists are so high and their criteria are so complex, by their lights few people can legitimately claim to be whole, and therefore well.

Mechanic (1978) points out that the concept of disease is being used with regard to nearly any kind of difficulty:

> When we apply the concept of disease to such conditions as pernicious anemia, syphilis, tuberculosis, and cancer, the underlying condition producing personal discomfort is relatively easily identified in terms of known clinical entities. However, when this concept is similarly applied to such conditions as neuroses, alcoholism, schizophrenia, and obesity, the basic roots of the problem may be much more ambiguous. When it is applied to such social problems as crime, suicide, political deviation, and illegitimacy, it becomes apparent that the concept of disease is widely applied but not always clearly formulated. (p. 25)

Indiscriminate use of the concept is a manifestation of the therapeutic culture described by Rieff (1968). Much of human activity is interpreted from a therapeutic perspective. Our language reflects this. Slow learners attend a reading "clinic." A lawbreaker is pronounced "sick." Unemployment is a "symptom" of economic "malaise." We even expect a "diagnosis" for car trouble.

The term "medicalization" has been used to describe the growing tendency to view many social problems from a therapeutic perspective (Crawford, 1980):

> Medicalization refers to the extension of the range of social phenomena mediated by the concepts of health and illness. . . . Alcoholism, child abuse, opiate addiction, obesity, problems with sexual functioning, and violence have all become matters for medical diagnosis, and the label of illness has been attached to them. (pp. 369–370)

Beaber (1983), who refers to this as "the diseasing of

America," suggests that our proclivity for turning difficulties into disorders serves the purpose of protecting us from the uncomfortable necessity of dealing with our own problems by exercising self-restraint. The label of disease allows us to abdicate responsibility to a caretaker. Beaber sketches a harsh parody of the "medicalized" individual:

> If a drunk driver kills my wife, how dare I hate him? We all know alcoholism is a disease and that no one gets a disease on purpose. But if I do hate him, if I'm out of my mind with rage and kill the driver, you can't be angry with me. After all, wasn't I suffering from temporary insanity? (That's a brief disease, like the flu). . . . Eating too much? That's OK, you're simply suffering from obesity. Certainly you needn't concern yourself with any lack of willpower. As we have all learned, your food problem is really just repressed sexuality, or maybe you don't have enough pineapple in your diet. . . . The one thing that is clear is that the problem isn't your fault and the solution could never be as simple as "Just stop eating so much." (p. 13)

Medicalization may be easy to scoff at in the version promoted by pop-psychologists, but its influence is pervasive. No less a figure than the surgeon general of the United States has suggested that violence is a health problem, treatable by physicians (Will, 1982).

We see illness everywhere. Almost any kind of disturbance can qualify us as sick; we need not have an obvious or measurable disorder. This is quite a contrast to Parsons's (1958) classic sick role. He named the primary criterion legitimizing assumption of this role as an incapacity for the effective performance of usual roles and tasks. Apple's (1960) research on how laymen define illness supports Parsons's concept. She concludes that, "to middle class Americans, to be ill means to have an ailment of recent origin which interferes with one's usual activities" (p. 223). In the culture of the therapeutic, one need not be unable to carry on activities as usual in order to be regarded as ill. One writer explains that "there are many people with no discernible physical illness, yet they feel bored, tense, anxious, or generally dissatisfied with their lives. This is not wellness although there is no classic illness" (Travis, 1980a, pp. 26). When boredom is an illness, the therapeutic culture has truly triumphed.

Apple also notes that "people with a high level of health care were more sensitive to the condition of interference with usual activities than were people with a low level of health care" (pp. 224–225). This suggests that the holistic concern with wellness may produce a certain hypochondria in those who take it seriously. Excessive concern with health may focus attention on minor discomforts that otherwise might have gone unnoticed, causing people to view with alarm every insignificant blip on their health-status screens. Pelletier (1979a) acknowledges this danger when he claims, "Paradoxical as it may seem, optimum health appears to occur only when an individual is no longer fixated upon whether it is present or not" (p. 21).

But Pelletier himself ignores the danger he speaks of when he claims that "at the present time, if an individual is deemed normal by medical or psychological examination, that means he is likely to become ill or die along with everyone else of comparable age, weight, and sex. This is certainly a dismal prognosis" (p. 16). The message here is that we are living in a fools' paradise if we measure ourselves against the standard of our peers. Medical evidence is limited, if not bogus. Only eternal vigilance will suffice. To be average is to be unwell.

For some, even wellness is not enough. Dunn (1961)

proposes that the ultimate health goal be considered "high-level wellness." This, he says, is a state in which movement occurs toward a higher functional potential, an open-ended future that offers challenges to meeting that potential, and complete integration of mind, body, spirit, and environment. According to this definition, individuals who are muddling along, feeling well and happy enough with their lot in life, but not meeting challenges that exercise their full potential are not really well. This kind of argument is itself sickening. It encourages people who are objectively well to be suspicious of their own sense of well-being. According to Thomas (1977), worry over personal health is a widespread problem:

> Nothing has changed so much in the health-care system over the past twenty-five years as the public's perception of its own health. The change amounts to a loss of confidence in the human form. The general belief these days seems to be that the body is fundamentally flawed, subject to disintegration at any moment, always on the verge of mortal disease, always in need of continual monitoring and support by health-care professionals. This is a new phenomenon in our society. (p. 43)

The holistic health movement must bear considerable responsibility for this change in our perceptions. By changing the norms for health and illness, it has produced what Bergsma and Thomasma (1982) call "normative dis-ease"—a disturbance in the way we experience our bodies that occurs when their realities fail to match socially established norms. The discrepancy between what our health status is and what the holists tell us it should be engenders feelings of anxiety, inadequacy, and guilt—or "dis-ease."

Even persons who qualify as healthy are warned that their status is tenuous. Baric (1969) suggests that individuals who engage in activities that significantly increase their risk for certain diseases, such as smoking and emphysema, assume an "at-risk" role, in which they are encouraged to recognize the relationship between their behavior and the potential for disease. Although this appears reasonable at first glance, it too has a sickening effect. How many among us, after all, behave in such a way that we never expose ourselves to risk? As Dubos points out, risk is inherent in life. People who are chronically anxious about their health may be less healthy than those who live with reckless abandon, enjoying all kinds of pleasures without regard to future consequences. As Paul Tillich states:

> Generally speaking, disease is a symptom of the universal ambiguity of life. Life must risk itself in order to win itself, but in the risking it may lose itself. A life which does not risk disease—even in the highest forms of the life of the spirit—is a poor life, as is shown, for instance, by the hypochondriac or the conformist. (1961, p. 94)

Further, the at-risk role implies that an objective set of behaviors exists that will contribute to health. Although this may be statistically true in some instances, (smokers *do* have a higher rate of lung cancer than nonsmokers), it ignores the phenomena of individuals who flaunt all the rules and appear the better for it.

And the rules become tougher all the time, growing more stringent as feeling good gives way to wellness, which in turn is replaced by high-level wellness. The result is that most of us meet the requirements of the at-risk role.

A further problem arises when we consider how difficult it is to measure wellness. If simply "feeling good" is no longer an acceptable criterion, and a physician's assessment is suspect, how are we to know if we are ill, well, high-level well, or at-risk? As Callan (1979) comments on "complete wellness" versus absence of illness: "Practitioners . . . [insist] that there is a distinct difference between the two. Perhaps there is, but it might be difficult to demonstrate a difference by objective, scientific means" (p. 1156).

Efforts have been made by conventional practitioners to establish measures of health and wellness. Breslow (1972), for example, tried to quantify the WHO definition. Parkerson et al. (1981) tested a health profile that measured four dimensions of health: symptom status, physical function, emotional function, and social function. Holists, too, have offered tools. Travis (1980c) devised a Wellness Inventory in which the person being evaluated received points for positive responses to the following statements.

> I keep an up-to-date record of my immunizations.
> My car gets at least 18 miles per gallon.
> I vote regularly.
> It is easy for me to laugh.
> I prepare my own baby food with a baby food grinder—
>   thus avoiding commercial foods. (pp. 145–146)

Behaviors deemed to constitute health risks vary among authors. But clearly, if not voting can threaten one's health, then the world is truly filled with risks. So, fearful that risk may evolve into active disease without our knowledge, we regularly present ourselves for testing in order to relieve our minds. But, as Horrobin points out, these procedures carry their own risks:

In contrast to its supposed benefits, screening may do considerable harm. . . . It subjects healthy people to a procedure which is worrying, no matter how well-informed they may be. It subtly creates an atmosphere in which people feel that no matter what their subjective sensations may be they may be unhealthy unless they have been screened and pronounced well. (1977, p. 36)

Screening, like much of what we do in the name of health, can contribute to our fretful self-absorption. Episodic health care is no longer enough. In conventional terms, patienthood is a status achieved by determining that one is ill and consulting a conventional provider (Eisenberg, 1980). One is no longer a patient when the illness is resolved. Holists prefer the role of "client," which appears to be something of a chronic condition. Ideally, clients see providers to learn what the threats to their health are and how to avoid them, a process that may be ongoing because the threats are so numerous. Indeed, the client may consult with a number of providers concurrently (psychotherapist, masseuse, nutritionist). Clienthood begins when people perceive themselves as vulnerable and in need of help to ward off perils. A picture in a holistic magazine bears the following caption: "The late Ida P. Rolf, Ph.D., creator of the Rolfing technique of structural integration, with a young client" (Smith, D., 1982, p. 21). The "client" appears to be about four months old. Clienthood, like other roles, is learned, and this child may be learning to feel unsafe in the world.

When we are encouraged to view ourselves "at-risk," how can we feel well? The sick role is expanding, the original Parsonian concept abandoned as hopelessly narrow. More people are sick, not because objective illness is increasing, but because it is becoming subjectively more difficult to feel well. It is ironic that the efforts of those holists who have popularized the notions of health promotion and illness prevention have contributed to the sickening of the populace.

Summary

The concept of health is losing its boundaries. Although individuals and groups have never precisely agreed as to what health is, and though the concept has changed markedly over time, until recently people could generally feel confident about whether or not they were ill. But changing ideas about health and illness have left us confused. It is now possible for individuals who feel strong as well as happy and who have no objective evidence of disease to be told that they are not well. As the definition of health has broadened, the possibilities for experiencing health have narrowed. Mattson (1982) believes that "the unattainability of the holistic concept of health is no problem to its advocates" (p. 11). It should be. Even though the holistic concept may represent a process, or an idealized goal, it has real consequences in the present.

It is crystallized in the slogan "Health is more than the absence of disease." What, in Scheffler's terms, is the value of this statement? It serves, as Mechanic noted, to indicate that other than purely physical factors may affect health. Given the weight of the evidence supporting the role of body-mind interactions in illness, it is a point well taken. We are not automatons functioning mechanically until we wind down or break down. In terms of literal accuracy, we might not question that health is more than the absence of disease.

We might, however, ask "how *much* more?" Is it really

mind, body, spirit, society, and environment functioning in total harmony? I think not. Health cannot be conceived of as something so large and complex that it is ultimately beyond our ability to be healthy. The holists have charged us with the responsibility to be healthy while creating a situation in which we cannot, thus causing frustration and anxiety. They have not succeeded in making us healthier, for health has been effectively priced out of the market. As a commodity, as something that can be achieved and maintained, it is further out of reach than ever.

4

The Individual

The focus of the holistic health movement is largely on the individual rather than society and its institutions. Although many writers acknowledge the influence of social and environmental influences on health, it is still the health of the individual that is of concern, rather than the health of groups. The movement has been criticized for its excessive concern with personal health (Crawford, 1980). When holists give consideration to larger arenas, it is usually for the purpose of pointing out the failure of some group or agency to offer protection to the individual. Institutional medicine, they say, cares only for its own profits and prestige as well as its ability to wield power. Hospitals and clinics are bureaucratic traps. Politicians strike compromises with business interests that allow them to foul the environment.

People are left to rely on themselves and what support is available from like-minded persons. They are frightened at the prospect of turning away from their doctors and the traditional health care they represent, but are driven to it by their anger at the faults they perceive: lack of caring, high cost, and ineffectiveness.

To the many among us who are similarly frightened, angered, and confused, the holistic health movement offers an alternative. It is not necessary, advocates say, to rely on others. Your health is—or can be—in your own hands. You can wrest control of it from the professionals; it is rightly yours. All persons, they believe, are most aware of their own health status and are therefore in the best position to direct, or even provide, their own health care. These responsibilities, once belonging to health-care professionals, now devolve on individuals. The patient role changes from one of passive recipient to one of greater responsibility and authority. As conventional medicine loses credibility, people are held increasingly accountable for managing their health-care activities. This chapter will consider the expectations that the holistic health movement has of the individual.

Prevention

Along with the promotion of health, the prevention of illness is seen as a primary goal of holistic health (Pelletier, 1979b). The traditional practice of treating disease after it has occurred is judged to be a less effective approach to health care than one that enables a person to avoid becoming ill in the first place. The holists are correct in suggesting that conventional medicine directs much of its energy toward treating illness. Yet there have always been practitioners with interest in preventive aspects of medicine.

Wain (1970) dates the beginning of the modern era of preventive medicine to Jenner's creation of a successful smallpox vaccine in 1796. During the next century, major advances were made in the prevention of communicable diseases, and at the turn of the century progress was made in the prevention of deficiency diseases. Rosen

(1977), tracing the growth of preventive medicine in the United States from 1900 to 1975, has noted the establishment of municipal and state health departments during the late 1800s and early 1900s. These departments were extensively involved in the diagnosis and control of communicable diseases. In 1899 the American Public Health Association established a Section on Bacteriology and Chemistry, and in 1909 the American Medical Association renamed one of its units the Section on Preventive Medicine and Public Health. These events were part of "a trend that developed with increased momentum in the first three decades of the present century, reflecting the widening scope and growing activism of the new public health based on expanding knowledge of disease prevention and health promotion" (p. 24).

According to Rosen, preventive medicine remained largely within the domain of public health and voluntary agencies during the first half of the century. Since then, he says, preventive health care has been increasingly incorporated into the clinical practices of individual providers; and the previous tendency to assign responsibility for prevention of disease to the agencies, with cure being within the domain of the practitioners, has diminished.

Supporting evidence for this claim can be seen in the growth of a number of clinical disciplines that emphasize preventive aspects of care. Nurse-midwives, for example, focus almost exclusively on preventing problems associated with childbearing. This is not to suggest that we are entering into a golden age of preventive health care; certainly, the interest of conventional providers in the more glamorous business of treating disease remains high. It does suggest, however, that holists may not claim an interest in preventing illness as their exclusive preserve.

Holists like to regard physicians as teachers whose job it is to instruct those under their care in behaviors that will prevent illness. It is a notion shared by others and can be found in ancient medical texts. The following is from *The Yellow Emperor's Classic of Internal Medicine* (circa 4th or 3rd century B.C.):

> The sages did not treat those who were already ill; they instructed those who were not yet ill. They did not want to rule those who were already rebellious; they guided those who were not yet rebellious. To administer medicines to diseases which have already developed and to suppress revolts which have already developed is comparable to the behaviour of those persons who begin to dig a well after they have become thirsty, and of those who begin to cast weapons after they have already engaged in battle. Would these actions not be too late? (in Veith, 1973, p. 18)

The holists would agree that treating manifest illness is an action taken too late. But they would not wish to rely on the sage-physician for preventive measures. The person at-risk must be involved as well. It is assumed that illness can be prevented if we undertake to engage in certain activities and avoid others. The holists can make a strong case that this is so. Much scientific evidence demonstrates that certain kinds of illness are related to behaviors potentially within the control of the individual.

It is known, for example, that most cases of liver cirrhosis are associated with excessive alcohol intake, that smokers have a much higher rate of lung cancer than nonsmokers, that scurvy does not afflict persons who ingest adequate amounts of vitamin C. A good deal of evidence supports the claim that cardiovascular status can be influenced by personal behavior. Noting the 21-percent decline in deaths from cardiovascular disease in the United States between 1968 and 1976, Goldman and Cook (1984) carefully reviewed the literature to determine how much of this decline was related to changes in life-style. They concluded that more than half the decrease in deaths could be attributed to reductions in cigarette smoking and fat consumption. Examples are too numerous to mention for which apparently simple preventive measures are known to medical science. (It is interesting to note the eagerness with which holists quote the conventional medical literature when it supports one of their theses.)

Lay persons, of course, would have difficulty trying to assimilate the massive amount of available data in such a way that they could make use of it. Traditionally, this has been a function performed by medical professionals, who have surveyed the evidence and advised us on what measures are indicated. It would be an overwhelming responsibility for the average person to try to sort this out. And confusion and disagreement exist even among professionals: witness the ongoing controversy surrounding the effects of dietary cholesterol. Preventive measures are aimed at reducing risk, and scientists do not always agree on the degree of risk inherent in a particular behavior. As indicated in the example given above, the weight of the scientific evidence indicates a high degree of risk associated with smoking.

In many instances, the degree of risk is less clear. Imperato and Mitchell (1985) describe the difficulty researchers have experienced in determining the association between tampon use and toxic shock syndrome (TSS): "If called upon to comment on the risks of TSS with tampon use most experts would say: We're sure, or almost sure, but perhaps not quite sure" (p. 149). Even those preventive measures that seem to offer genuine benefits sometimes carry their own price, as attested to by the numerous orthopedic complaints of runners.

The bewildered individual who turns for guidance to the holistic literature is likely to become even more confused. The prescriptions for diet, activity, medication, exercise, and life-style are numerous and often contradictory. Do I need more zinc in my diet? Less fat? Which stress-reducing techniques should I use? How many kinds of exercise are required for total fitness? The person who seriously pursued answers to these kinds of questions would find it necessary to make the quest for health a kind of quasi-career. Indeed, many people do get caught up in this kind of "healthism."

The holists have responded to this criticism by suggesting that multiple therapies are required because each person is unique and will respond to a particular treatment or variety of treatments that might be ineffective for another person. It is believed necessary for individuals to find their own ways to health. Standard protocols that do not consider this uniqueness are not likely to achieve a therapeutic effect.

Although the argument that response to treatment varies with the individual certainly contains much truth, the likelihood of a positive response can be established. Medical science is in part based on probabilities. That is, it can be determined what my chances of contracting measles are following vaccination, but I cannot be guaranteed that I will not develop measles. Therapeutic effect of a given treatment may be determined by the trial-and-error method using large populations, making it unnecessary for each person to conduct his or her own trials. It would certainly seem to be more reliable and less exhausting to have the efficacy of procedures determined in this way. True, we all have our notions about what works for us in the prevention of colds, stiff necks, and other ills, and it is likely, based on research with placebos, that our beliefs will influence the outcome. Too, physiological differences exist among people that affect response to preventive measures. Nevertheless, these variables need not eliminate the use of protocols that may then be tailored to the individual.

A number of protocols for preventive health care have been established. In *Healthy People: The Surgeon General's Report on Health Promotion and Disease Prevention* (U.S. Department of Health, Education, and Welfare, 1979), lay people are advised on a number of preventive measures as well as those for the early detection of disease. Recommendations include such items as daily brushing and flossing of teeth, yearly dental exams, regular exercise, and wise use of alcohol. Frame (1986) has formulated a protocol for health maintenance to be used by physicians that focuses on screening for particular problems. He compares his recommendations to those made by the Canadian Task Force on the Periodic Health Examination and those of the American Cancer Society. Similarities exist among the three groups in many items, but a number of differences are apparent as well. Berg (1986) comments as follows on Frame's analysis: "Virtually every recommendation is arguable in some dimension" (p. 319). As yet, health professionals do not absolutely agree as to what constitutes the ideal preventive regimen. Nevertheless, agreement is sufficient on a number of issues to provide some guidance to the lay person on prudent health behavior.

Sometimes, however, scientific knowledge about disease prevention is ignored or poorly communicated to the public. The epidemic of acquired immunodeficiency syndrome (AIDS) offers an instructive example. We now have solid evidence that many cases of AIDS are potentially preventable by individual behavioral changes related to drug use and sexual activity (Francis and Chin, 1987). Nevertheless, some people continue to engage in high-risk behaviors, such as sharing unsterile needles and engaging in unprotected sexual intercourse with multiple partners. And, although casual and household contact has *not* been documented as a means of transmission of human immunodeficiency virus (HIV), we continue to see reports in the press of children being kept out of school by fearful parents (Levine, J., 1986).

It is particularly interesting to observe that prevention has a twofold aspect with this syndrome. First, as just noted, there must be concern about transmission of the virus; and second, those who are already infected with HIV become concerned with preventing the actual development of AIDS. Although no effective means of preventing AIDS in persons with HIV infection has been documented, this group is particularly vulnerable to the promises of "holistic" or "alternative" therapies. Thus, some persons with AIDS-related complex, as well as those with AIDS, have resorted to purchasing unapproved drugs and engaging in such treatments as ingesting processed pond scum or striking the chest "to stimulate the thymus gland" (Monmaney, 1987).

The holistic petition for "whatever works" does remind us that people are unpredictable and must be treated as individuals. No one treatment will work for everyone. A person's own preventive regimen may change over time. Elderly people, for example, may find that they must take better measures to protect themselves from extremes in temperature in order to avoid becoming ill. But the holists must offer some guidelines. It is not enough to suggest that each individual invent a personal regimen. I would not deny a person that which "works" for him or her, but we need to know further what preventive measures work best for most people. I cannot do everything recommended by everyone; that would exhaust me physically, emotionally, and financially, leaving me no time to live my life (and very possibly ill besides).

What can I reasonably be expected to do to protect my health? Some holists have recognized the importance of this question and have sought to provide an answer. They offer a more modest and more reasonable approach than those who advocate multiple therapies. It is their contention that a few simple health rules, if followed faithfully, will lead to greatly improved health. The research conducted by Belloc and Breslow (1972) is frequently cited. They identify seven behaviors that significantly influence health: (1) eating breakfast; (2) eating regular meals without snacking; (3) maintaining normal weight for height; (4) not smoking cigarettes; (5) drinking alcohol moderately, if at all; (6) exercising at least moderately; and (7) sleeping seven to eight hours per night. It was found that the effect of maintaining these habits was cumulative, that is, people who followed four were healthier than those who followed three; those who followed five were healthier than those who followed four, etc. Furthermore, life expectancy increased as the number of habits increased (Belloc, 1973).

LaLonde (1980) suggests that lack of absolute certainty about the cause of illness should not deter us from pursuing seemingly reasonable courses of action. Therefore, although we do not clearly understand the effects of obesity or exercise on health, we should proceed on the assumption that "it is better to be slim than fat" and "exercise and fitness are better than sedentary living and lack of fitness" (p. 451). If by "better" LaLonde means "healthier," his argument is worth considering.

Health professionals are continually impressed by the

poor health of those who fail to follow the kind of commonsense health rules advocated by Belloc and Breslow, LaLonde, and others. Empirically, it is hard to deny the wisdom of the precept "Moderation in all things." The effects of smoking, overeating, and alcohol abuse are particularly apparent and grievous. Nurses and doctors caring for those suffering from emphysema, coronary artery disease, and cirrhosis of the liver must at times sadly conclude, as the holists do, that the person's own behavior was the cause. Particularly troubling is the fact that such behavior is likely to continue even following repeated warnings of the consequences. It is a frustrating experience to spend many dollars and much time and energy nursing patients back to health after an illness, only to have them leave the hospital, resume their old habits and return, perhaps even sicker than before. Some patients, chafing under the restrictions of, say, a low-sodium diet, even openly cheat or announce their intentions to do so upon returning home.

This problem, known as "noncompliance," is largely ignored by the holists, though an extensive body of research on it is available in the conventional health-care literature. Noncompliance (failure to follow a therapeutic regimen recommended by a health-care provider) is a problem of serious proportions. In studies involving long-term or preventive regimens, or when the patient is asymptomatic, noncompliance averages about 50 percent (Becker, M. H., 1979). Those who espouse the approach of living by simple health rules seem to believe that, if people simply understand the benefits to be gained, they would soon change their ways. Pelletier (1979a) acknowledges that, "though the concept of prevention is relatively easy, its implementation is problematic" and claims that behavior can be changed by providing a "sustained intelligible message which is reinforced by peer pressure and results in clearly perceived rewards in a relatively short period of time" (p. 10). The difficulty is that peer pressure is often lacking or working at cross-purposes, and rewards may not be evident for years. Even then, they may be framed in negative terms: "I have not had a stroke." The provider is then left with the hope that a "sustained intelligible message," that is, patient education, will be enough.

It is a naive hope. As Milio (1976) points out, if knowledge of healthful practices were sufficient, health providers themselves would be models of healthy behavior. In some instances, simply providing information about a health risk does lead to a change in behavior. In a study conducted by telephone interviews, 45 percent of persons who regarded themselves as at-risk for genital herpes said they had modified their sexual behavior to decrease the possibility of contracting the disease (Aral, Cates, and Jenkins, 1985).

On the whole, however, research does not indicate a strong relationship between knowledge and compliance (Matthews and Hingson, 1977). A case in point is a study of families with children who had been prescribed a ten-day course of penicillin. The families' knowledge about the disease and its treatment was high: 80 percent had an adequate knowledge of the diagnosis, 90 percent knew the medication being used was penicillin, and 95 percent understood the correct directions for administration. In spite of this high level of knowledge, however, at least 82 percent of the children had stopped receiving the drug by the ninth day of treatment (Bergman and Werner, 1963).

Eventually, the holists will be forced to come to terms with what the conventional providers already know: most people "fail to comply" for reasons other than lack of information. Among the less sophisticated holists, this comes as a tremendous surprise because they themselves are likely to modify their behavior in order to improve their health. Some are cheerily unaware that anything so "simple" as healthy behavior can be difficult or impossible to achieve. Others are hurt or even angered at what they see as irresponsible behavior. These are responses generated by a simple view of a complicated phenomenon.

Healthy behavior, however, is anything but simple. Haynes (1982) notes that not only has little success been achieved in studies using patient education as the single intervention to increase compliance, but also that more than 250 other factors have been positively associated with compliance. "As a result, simple theories, such as 'the patient is ignorant' have been found wanting" (p. 56). Among the factors that have been discovered to be associated with compliance are the quality of the patient-provider relationship (Matthews and Hingson, 1977), the psychological utility of the behavior to be altered (Horn, 1976), and the simplicity of the therapeutic regimen (Reichgott and Simmons-Morton, 1983).

According to Rosenstock (1966), health behavior is closely related to the beliefs of individuals about how susceptible they are to a particular problem, how serious the problem is, and the relative costs and benefits of taking remedial action. Rosenstock's model has been tested extensively. Each of the factors he identifies has been related to the probability that an individual will adopt particular health behaviors (Mikhail, 1981).

Although research has provided some insights into health behavior, to date no one has devised a sure and simple means of assuring that individuals will actually practice health-promoting behavior. Surely the holists are right in assuming that poor personal health habits result in much illness and suffering, and we must share the hope that it need not be so. As Breslow (1977) observes, poor health habits *can* be changed, though the resistance to change is strong. The holists would make a significant contribution if they could enlarge our understanding of why well-informed people continue self-destructive behavior patterns.

It cannot be assumed, however, that illness can be prevented solely by individual initiative. Epidemiology has not reached the point where an exact cause can be identified for every illness, nor do we have the means to prevent every disease for which a cause is known. In the first instance, multiple sclerosis remains a mystery; in the second, narrow-angle glaucoma can be treated, but not always prevented. At times, when we think we know how to prevent illness, our means are inadequate. Even individuals who receive recommended vaccinations can (very rarely) develop polio, and a low incidence of lung cancer exists among nonsmokers. That is not to suggest that we start smoking or neglect vaccinations, but to point out that no method is fail-safe.

Some health problems are beyond the individual's power to prevent. Environmental hazards, such as air pollution, acid rain, and toxic waste, are clearly beyond the influence of a single person. Even those aspects discussed previously that are seemingly within the control of the individual may be placed out of reach by social and political constraints. A single mother of three young children who is living in poverty might find it impossible to get enough sleep or eat a good diet; she probably wouldn't deem exercise to be a high priority. It has been pointed out that holism, in focusing on the individual, may prevent us from recognizing and acting on some of the social causes of illness (Berliner and Salmon, 1980).

One argument that is frequently used in support of increasing health-promotion/disease-prevention activities is that they constitute a good economic investment. Holists and others assure us that an ounce of prevention really is worth a pound of cure. And, in fact, promotion/ prevention programs have increased rapidly in numbers in recent years. Higgins (1986) asserts that the force behind these programs in both the public and private sectors is a desire to control rising health-care costs. It would seem to make common sense that efforts to maintain health today would lead to savings on disease treatment in the future. This is the belief of Joseph Califano, who points out that in 1984 the United States spent less than 1 percent of its $112 billion health-care budget on promotion/prevention (1986).

If we were to spend more money, would we actually realize larger savings? The answer is not clear. Warner (1987) describes a number of flaws in the conventional wisdom that promotion/prevention dollars spent inevitably result in treatment dollars saved. First, he observes that some costs associated with health-promotion programs are only apparent years after the program has been offered, and may be overlooked. He cites the example of smoking-cessation programs, some of which are very successful. Although they may cut employer costs for such items as sick leave and health insurance, Warner notes that they can add to firms' pension costs by increasing the number of years former smokers survive after retirement.

Warner also suggests that those evaluating the outcomes of health-promotion programs may mistakenly assume that the desired change in behavior (smoking cessation, for example) leads to a corresponding change in risk. In fact, he says, though the mortality of ex-smokers drops sharply after the habit is stopped, it does not approximate that of persons who have never smoked for at least fifteen years. Finally, Warner suggests that "knowledge of the long-term effectiveness of most health promotion programs is relatively primitive" (p. 50). Thus, calculating savings attributable to these programs is difficult.

Also contributing to this difficulty is the fact that not all the potential benefits of prevention/promotion activities can be assigned a monetary value. Although holists may try to sell programs to government and private interests on the basis of cost-savings, some programs may have outcomes that are useful to the individual participant, but not necessarily financially rewarding to the sponsoring agency. According to Engleman and Forbes (1986), programs may have both investment value and consumption value. The investment value can, at least in theory, be measured by looking at the dollar savings stimulated by a program. Consumption value, on the other hand, cannot be measured in economic terms. It is the nonmonetary value that can be placed on good health and the freedom that it affords the individual to lead a full and satisfying life free of unnecessary pain, suffering, and disability.

Consumption values related to health are certainly not to be underestimated, and holists concentrate heavily on them, emphasizing such vague outcomes as "wellness." However, advocating a program that is likely to produce mainly consumption value as cost-saving is misleading. Do the holists produce much in the way of investment value? Certainly some preventive measures have investment value—fluoridating the water supply has substantially reduced the cost of treating dental caries—but this is not something that the holists can take credit for. Nor can they take credit for any of the other major preventive successes of public health, such as the decrease in the incidence of certain communicable diseases by immunization. To date, the holists have not succeeded in

demonstrating that they have been successful in pro-
ducing cost-savings through the use of health-promotion
activities. Thus, the economic argument is not impressive.

Responsibility

Closely related to the concept of prevention is that of
responsibility. And, "You are responsible for your own
health" is one of the holistic slogans that has gained the
widest recognition and acceptance outside of the movement. If we assume that many illnesses can be prevented
by an act of will or by certain kinds of behavior, then it
is easy to conclude that people ought to think and behave
in these ways. Individuals are seen as having a measure
of control over whether or not they become ill. They are
responsible for their own health:

> Health and disease don't just happen to us. They are
> active processes issuing from inner harmony or dishar-
> mony, profoundly affected by our states of conscious-
> ness, our ability or inability to flow with experience. This
> recognition carries with it implicit responsibility and op-
> portunity. If we are participating, however uncon-
> sciously, in the process of disease, we can choose health
> instead. (Ferguson, M., 1980, p. 257)

This statement indicates that the holistic understanding of personal responsibility for health goes far beyond
the scope of conventional preventive practices. The message here is not simply that we should avoid known disease-causing agents and activities. Ferguson intends us
to understand that illness is not simply a physical event
occasioned by an attack from something in the environ-

ment over which we have no control. Rather, it is a phenomenon in which the person chooses, in some way, to
become vulnerable.

Common sense informs us that certain practices—say
eating a diet of junk food—may cause us to become ill.
The holistic concept of responsibility for health includes
this understanding, but goes further. Whereas medical
descriptions of disease causation have a physiological
bias, holistic explanations have a psychological bias. Holists differ only in the degree to which they believe psychological phenomena influence illness. Health and
illness are related not only to what we do or do not do,
but to what we think, how we feel, even who we are.
This follows from the cardinal tenet of mind-body-spirit
unity. In spite of the emphasis on unity, many holists
give first billing to the mental component:

> The state of health is defined by a personal belief system
> which is in accordance with physiological and genetic
> endowments. Health is the absence of disease, a state of
> balance that is accomplished through harmonious energy
> which in turn actualizes loving thought habits towards
> oneself and others. A block in this harmonious flow of
> energy always precedes disease and illness. This in turn
> inhibits the body's natural tendency towards dynamic
> equilibrium. (Taub, 1983, p. 3)

The self may be a unity of body, mind, and spirit, but,
to the holist, the mind is first among equals.

The difficult questions surrounding the issue of the
influence of the mind on health has been distilled down
to a simplistic formula: the wrong feelings, or any feelings handled in the wrong way, can make you ill. This
has become a piece of received wisdom that is passed
along quite casually. In an article in a news magazine

on men's seeming inability to establish intimate relationships, one writer said, "Men nurture their feelings
only inwardly and later harvest ulcers or heart attacks"
(Engel, E., 1982, p. 13).

The above interpretation represents a popularization
of the specificity theory that was formulated by the psychosomatic branch of medicine. Although the study of
psychosomatics includes all features of mind-body relationships, one aspect of early and continuing interest
was specificity theory, or the relationship between specific emotions, attitudes, or personality characteristics
and the onset of disease. Dunbar (1947–48), whose work
in psychosomatics is regarded as seminal, claims that
"the tendency of certain types of personality to acquire
certain types of heart disease is marked, but it should be
applied to any given individual only with a great many
reservations" (p. 130).

Even before the establishment of psychosomatic medicine as a specialty, some diseases were described as having specific psychic antecedents. Many physicians in the
eighteenth and nineteenth centuries were convinced that
cancer could be occasioned by an attitude of hopelessness and despair following trauma or loss (Kowal, 1955).
And, for many years, particular personality types have
been associated with certain disorders: ulcerative colitis—" . . . extremely hard to please, very dependent,
immature, apathetic, and hypercritical of anything and
everything that is done for them" (De Luca, 1970, p. 23);
chronic gastric ulcer—" . . . personality pattern of independence and self-sufficiency . . . prone to anxiety
and depression" (Alp, Court, and Grant, 1970, p. 773);
tension headache—" . . . rather rigid, compulsive and
perfectionistic" (Martin, 1966, p. 51).

Descriptions of the personality type associated with a
particular disorder often vary. Shapiro and Goldstein

note that "for more than 40 years, personality traits have been linked with hypertensive disorders. Nevertheless, we are still unable to specify which personality factors relate to hypertension. For each study relating hypertension to a particular personality pattern, there is another exhibiting contradictory or negative results" (1982, p. 843). Here, the question of cause and effect must be raised. If these descriptions are accurate, does that imply that the personality characteristics caused the health problem? In the case of the "migraine personality," Blaszczynski (1984) suggests that the supposedly typical traits of hostility, obsessiveness, neuroticism, and anxiety may be the result, not the cause, of headache pain.

Specificity theory is not universally supported by psychosomatic researchers. A five-year study of 187 adults failed to demonstrate that psychosomatic disorders appear in a single body system in a given individual. Instead, diffuse manifestations of psychosomatic disease occurred (Buck and Hobbs, 1965). Alexander, reviewing the literature on emotional aspects of asthma, concluded that, though "psychological variables would be potentially important for some asthmatics some of the time," the research to date does not support a psychological etiology for this disease (1981, p. 333). Ader (1980) points out that, though many studies have established a relationship between disease and psychosocial factors, the relative contributions of these factors to susceptibility to disease has not been established, particularly with regard to individuals.

Galdston (1965) has described two errors sometimes made by psychosomatic investigators. The first he calls the error of specificity. This is the assumption that every psychosomatic disease has a specific psychic cause. The second is the fallacy of time-sequence causality, which involves the assumption that if B follows A, then B is caused by A. Holists frequently make both of these errors when interpreting findings from the psychosomatic literature. They may fail to recognize that a psychic factor represents only one variable in the etiology of an illness. This and the tendency to confuse correlation with causation contribute to the holists' beliefs that disease is largely a psychic phenomenon, potentially under the control of the individual.

Stress is the generalized culprit, felt to be a contributor to almost any disease imaginable. An enormous and impressive literature illustrates a significant relationship between stress and disease. Research in this area is particularly vulnerable to faulty interpretation involving the errors described by Galdston. A case in point is the body of studies relating disease and the stress experienced by an individual who experiences many life changes in a brief period of time.

Many studies have demonstrated a relationship between life events and specific physical problems such as menstrual discomfort (Siegel, Johnson, and Sarason, 1979), recurrent herpes labialis (Schmidt, Zyzanski, Ellner, Kumar, and Arno, 1985), and myocardial infarction (Connolly, 1976). Not all such studies have shown a positive relationship, however. An investigation using several measures of stress, including one that measured life change, failed to demonstrate that stress predisposes a woman to breast cancer (Priestman, Priestman, and Bradshaw, 1985). Another study reported a *negative* correlation between recent life events and the complications of pregnancy (Jones, 1978). Given such negative findings, we must refrain from concluding that every type of physical problem is related to life changes.

That many physical problems *are* related to the stress of life changes, however, is undeniable. A key problem to analyze is the precise nature of that relationship.

Dohrenwend and Dohrenwend, veterans of several decades of research in the field, state the problem clearly:

> Up to now the overwhelming number of studies of life stress and illness have simply asked: does life stress relate to changes in health? Since the answer to this question is clearly affirmative, we can now move on to the question: how does life stress relate to changes in health? (1984, p. 22)

It is tempting to conclude that life change *causes* illness. Connolly, however, cautions against assuming a cause-effect relationship: "It may be that some pre-illness behavior is causing both disease and events and that the events themselves are irrelevant to the cause" (1976, p. 12). Here we see the possibility of committing the time-sequence causality fallacy. The answer to the Dohrenwends' question is not so simple as A causes B. Wershow and Reinhart, in fact, suggest that, though life change and illness are related, "the relationship is a weak one" (1974, p. 400). Further research may indeed reveal a causal relationship between life change and some diseases, but at present no such relationship has been established.

The error of specificity is often made by those who subscribe to the notion that particular ways of handling emotions are pathogenic. It has been suggested that the inhibition of expression of all kinds of emotions is an important cause of psychosomatic diseases (Groen, 1974). Unexpressed anger, in particular, is regarded as dangerous. It has been associated with such disorders as hypertension (Gentry, Chesney, Gary, Hall, and Harburg, 1982) and rheumatoid arthritis (Cobb, 1959). Cancer is the prototype disease of this kind. The typical cancer patient has been described as someone who is supportive of others but is quietly despairing inwardly and is unable to express negative feelings (LeShan, 1977). The repressed emotions will not be denied, and eventually find expression in the form of cancer.

Susan Sontag has attacked this notion, noting that a similar etiology was ascribed to tuberculosis before the cause (a bacillus, not an emotion) was identified: "Doctors and laity believed in a TB character type—as now the belief in a cancer-prone character type, far from being confined to the back yard of folk superstition, passes for the most advanced medical thinking" (1979, p. 38). It is not an accident that holists have been particularly attracted to cancer as an exemplar of the influence of emotions. The failure of medicine to determine a precise etiology has allowed nonphysical explanations to flourish. As Sontag says, "Theories that diseases are caused by mental states and can be cured by will power are always an index of how much is not understood about the physical terrain of a disease" (p. 54).

Altering the Course of Disease

When we do become ill, the holists expect us to harness our emotions in the service of becoming well. They enjoy pointing to the celebrated case of Norman Cousins, who, after being diagnosed with ankylosing spondylitis (a serious degenerative disease of connective tissue in the spine), embarked on a self-treatment program with the blessing of his physician. It involved removing himself from the hospital to a hotel room, stopping his prescribed medication regimen, taking huge amounts of vitamin C intravenously, and dosing himself periodically with laughter via tapes of the old "Candid Camera" TV show.

Cousins made a recovery viewed as remarkable by his physicians.

Every ingredient of this drama lends itself to a holistic interpretation. The patient defies all the rules of the medical establishment and wins! He, not the doctor, is in charge; he absconds to a less treacherous environment; the "toxic" drugs are replaced with a "natural" one. Most important, he uses his emotions to reverse the disease process:

> The inevitable question arose in my mind: what about the positive emotions? If negative emotions produce negative chemical changes in the body, wouldn't the positive emotions produce positive changes? Is it possible that love, hope, faith, laughter, confidence and the will to live have therapeutic value? (1981, pp. 34–35).

Cousins's recovery is touted as evidence that the emotions can be used to regain health.

For those who believe that psychic factors can cause disease, it seems a logical next step to conclude that psychic factors can cure or control disease. This is the belief of the Simontons (1980), whose work with terminally ill cancer patients is based on the premise that even very ill people can markedly affect their health using the powers of the mind. They state that cancer patients participating in their program, which includes relaxation techniques and visualization exercises, have lived 1 1/2 to 2 times longer than expected. In particular, the Simontons believe that feelings of helplessness and hopelessness need to be altered if cancer patients are to improve their chances of survival.

In a prospective study of seriously ill cancer patients, however, Cassileth, Lusk, Miller, Brown, and Miller (1985) found that psychosocial factors, including the degree of hopelessness/helplessness, were *not* predictive of length of survival. In another study, investigators were surprised to find that patients who reported requiring the most psychological adjustment in terms of coping with malignant melanoma were least likely to experience a relapse. They concluded that "these data suggest that if the illness has progressed too far, psychological factors may not be related to survival any longer" (Rogentine, van Kammen, Fox, Docherty, Rosenblatt, Boyd, and Bunney, 1979, p. 652).

Correlational studies such as these can provide information about the relationship between emotions and disease. They do not, however, say anything about the possibility of altering that relationship. Is it true, as some practitioners claim, that we can actually alter the course of disease by psychic means? Two studies involving Type A behavior were unsuccessful in establishing that health outcomes could be influenced by altering behavioral traits. Friedman and Rosenman describe Type A individuals as "doers" who have a high level of time urgency. They have a strong need for achievement, are often involved with many activities requiring deadlines, and tend to think and move rapidly. Type B individuals, on the other hand, do not exhibit these traits. Friedman and Rosenman (1959) found that men who exhibited Type A behavior were seven times more likely than Type B individuals to have evidence of clinical coronary artery disease. However, in a study by Suinn and Bloom (1978), subjects who received anxiety management training for three weeks showed a decrease in anxiety and Type A behavior, but no decrease in blood pressure, cholesterol, or triglycerides—all factors associated with cardiovascular disease.

In another study, post-myocardial infarction patients were provided with (1) counseling on changing Type A behavior; or (2) Type A counseling and cardiac counseling, including information on diet, exercise, risk factors, etc.; or (3) no counseling. Subjects receiving both Type A counseling and cardiac counseling significantly modified their Type A behavior. Their risk for cardiac recurrence was significantly lower than for subjects receiving no counseling, but was *not* significantly lower than for those receiving only cardiac counseling (Powell, Friedman, Thoreson, Gill, and Ulmer, 1984). These studies indicate that, though individuals can alter Type A behavior, doing so will not necessarily decrease the risk of heart disease.

The holists ask us to prevent or alter the course of disease by manipulating our emotional responses. This may or may not be effective. But, if we accept for the moment that it is, if I change those personal characteristics which caused me to get, for example, heart disease, might I not simply be making myself vulnerable to another kind of disease? If overt expressions of hostility are associated with heart disease and repression of hostility with cancer, does that mean people must choose which disease they would rather risk? It is interesting to note that the emotions and personality characteristics associated with disease are all negative: anxiety, hostility, depression, etc. One wonders what diseases might be statistically related to cheerfulness, humor, and hope. What does the well-adjusted person die of?

The Limits of Personal Responsibility for Health

How should we evaluate the statement "You are responsible for your own health"? On the commonsense "be sure to brush your teeth" level, we can safely assume that we must accept responsibility. Can we go further and believe, as the holists ask us to do, that responsibility extends to the way we handle our emotions—that as the Simontons say: "Everyone participates in his or her health or illness at all times"? (1980, p. 3) The fact that illness is at times statistically associated with emotional factors is not in doubt. The person seeking to understand the meaning of the statistical association, however, will not find consensus or clarity in the literature.

Note the differences between the following statements on holistic medicine:

> On the basis of an exhaustive review of the literature relating cancer to stressful psychological experiences, for example, one expert has concluded that stresses specific to the individual might contribute about 10% to the start of cancers in individuals aged 40 to 60. . . . If the data are correct, the only legitimate conclusion is that the part played by emotional factors in the onset of cancer is relatively small compared with genetic vulnerabilities and environmental carcinogens (Frank, 1981, p. 226).

> The key to being well is mental health. Mentally well-adjusted individuals have only 10% of the serious illness rate of maladjusted individuals. . . . We are in control of 90% of the things that shorten our lives (Siegel and Siegel, 1981, p. 442).

The figures quoted in the two statements are referring to different things and cannot be compared. But each author clearly represents opposite sides of the emotion-illness controversy. No agreement prevails on the issue, and "facts" are trotted out to support both sides. Emotional factors are highly correlated with some diseases in particular, but correlation does not prove causation. Even if causation were to be demonstrated, that would not provide conclusive evidence that disease which was caused by emotions could have been prevented or could be cured by emotions handled differently. Those holists who claim that this is so take the evidence far beyond what it is able to support. According to Angell, much evidence relating physical disease with mental state is anecdotal, and scientific studies are frequently seriously flawed. "The evidence for mental state as a cause and cure of today's scourges is not much better than it was for the afflictions of earlier centuries" (1985, p. 1571).

The truth is that, though we know that mind and body influence one another, we are just beginning to learn how this works; we know even less about how it can be controlled. It is naive at best to assume that we have complete psychic control of our health. Yet, this is the dangerous notion being promulgated by some. One physician goes so far as to suggest that our control extends even to death. The following statement is included in a "bill of rights" he provides to cancer patients: "Do not tell me how long I have to live. I alone can decide how long I will live. It is my desires, my goals, my values, my strengths, and my will to live that will make the decision" (Siegel and Siegel, 1981, p. 441).

Although some notable successes have been achieved in treating some physical ailments, such as hypertension, with psychological therapies (Benson, 1975), it would be naive to expect that all disorders would be similarly responsive to such treatment. We have been wrong before when describing the etiology of illness as psychological. Kopelman and Moskop (1981) point out the particularly unfortunate example of childhood autism, which was at one time blamed on overly demanding and unaffectionate parents. It is now regarded as congenital. And stories have appeared in the lay press advising the public that "you can stop feeling guilty about your ulcer. It has nothing to do with your personality or your diet—it's a biological disease" (Caldwell, 1983, p. 34).

The holistic charge to "be responsible" is itself irresponsible when it goes beyond what is known about our ability to comply. I cannot be responsible for that which I cannot control, and it is not yet clear, beyond a certain point, how far that control extends. Norman Cousins himself warns that "it is manifestly true that interest in these matters outruns systematic knowledge" (1981, p. 117). Two flawed (or at least unproven) beliefs are apparent in the holistic scheme of self-responsibility: first, that all illness is primarily psychological in origin; second, that the individual can control or prevent it by mental maneuvers. Insofar as the holists base their understanding of health and illness on these beliefs, I cannot accept the responsibility they say is mine. At the most, holists may claim, "You are in some circumstances, and to some degree, responsible for your own health."

Guilt

When health is held among the highest of values and is believed to be a state achievable by right acts and sufficient will, illness ceases to be a misfortune and is taken as evidence of moral failing. To be responsible for my health means minimally that I have some influence over it. To the holists, it means that I am obligated to exercise that influence. If I do not, I will fall ill, and my illness will expose my lack of responsibility. Health is no longer just to be desired, it is required of the upright person; it is not something to be enjoyed, but something to be produced. How different this is from the more typical view described by Engelhardt:

> Health is a normative concept but not in the sense of a moral virtue. Though health is a good, and though it may be morally praiseworthy to try to be healthy and to advance the health of others, still, all things being equal, it is a misfortune, not a misdeed, to lack health. Health is more an aesthetic than an ethical term; it is more beauty than virtue. Thus, one does not condemn someone for no longer being healthy, though one may sympathize with him over the loss of a good. (1981, p. 31)

Holists take the exactly opposite position. Health has much to do with rectitude. Although adherents may deny it, the holistic health movement is greatly concerned with good and bad behavior regarding health. And, because health is defined in such a way as to include almost everything, the movement has an essentially moralistic stance toward human activity in general. Mechanic (1978) observes that deviant behavior is often evaluated from either a "health-illness" perspective or a "goodness-badness" perspective. Assignment of a particular behavior to either the "sick" or "bad" category is an arbitrary decision influenced not only by the behavior itself, but also by a number of social factors. However, "most physical illnesses (deviations from medically derived standards of normal functioning) fall within definitions of 'sickness' rather than 'badness' " (p. 50).

Not so to the holist. Physical illness is believed to carry a message to the victim that something is amiss in his or her way of life:

Are you responsible for the cold? Yes, at some level you are. You may have no conscious awareness of it, but you created the condition which weakened your body and made it an environment of "dis-ease." If you are self-responsible, you will accept the cold as an important message from your body, and use it as a chance to rest and rebalance. (Ryan and Travis, 1981, p. 12)

Contrary to Mechanic's statement, the holists do not remove physical illness from the badness category. And, as discussed in the last chapter, many nonphysical deviations are defined as illness. The holistic classification of a particular behavior as bad or sick, in fact, is often directly opposed to the conventional assignment. Drug abuse, once regarded as bad or criminal, is now something to be treated, whereas heart disease may be viewed as the inevitable result of a self-indulgent life-style.

Physical illness has become suspect. The burden of proof is on the individual to demonstrate that he or she has not "participated" in the illness. The obligations attending illness have changed, too. Formerly, the Parsonian sick role required only that the person try to get better, usually by seeking professional help: "He is not expected to make himself better by 'good motivation' or high resolve without the help of others" (Fox, R. C., 1977, p. 15). These are precisely the requirements of the holistic sick role. The sick person has behaved badly and will have to make reparations.

This message is delivered sometimes earnestly and with professed compassion for the sick, and sometimes with a smug, self-righteous tone. In either case, the message is the same: He who is sick must bear the blame. It is an instance of "blaming-the-victim" (Crawford, 1980) and, as with the rape victim, there are subtle or not so

subtle implications that the victim was "asking for it."
It is frequently suggested that people use illness to meet
unacknowledged psychological needs in an acceptable
manner:

> Illness has always been an acceptable excuse for not
> going to school or work. And cancer is the current
> "heavy-duty" permission to avoid returning to a stressful
> job, and a legitimate reason for even the toughest person
> to ask for help and attention. People whose lives have
> been ineffectual or lonely may discover that having can-
> cer gives them the kind of personal power and attention
> they have always wanted. (Fiore, 1979, p. 288)

Fiore is telling us that cancer speaks for its victims, expressing what they are unable to say themselves. This is
what Sontag (1979) is talking about when she says, "The
view of cancer as a disease of the failure of expressiveness
condemns the cancer patient: expresses pity but also con-
veys contempt" (p. 47).

Contempt *is* implicit in the holistic formulation of personal responsibility, and it is one of the ugliest manifestations of the movement. The idea that the patient is
blameworthy has created a great deal of suffering for
many, and the movement has been soundly criticized for
it (Shapiro and Shapiro, 1979; Glickman, 1979). People
who truly believe that they are responsible for their
health will necessarily feel guilt upon becoming ill. They
will feel that they "had it coming to them."

Many in the movement, well aware of this criticism,
have desperately tried to defend themselves against it
by trying to disassociate the concepts of "responsibility"
and "blame":

Taking responsibility for choices which result in illness does not mean taking on blame. There is a big difference. With blame you berate yourself for not learning a lesson, or burden yourself with guilt which creates more stress. With responsibility, you accept that you engineered your life situation, and that you can change it as well. (Ryan and Travis, 1981, p. 12)

This is a facile argument that attempts to explain away the difficulties inherent in holistic responsibility. By redefining blame and guilt, the holists are ducking their own accountability for having created guilt and unhappiness with their creed. At any rate, the distinction between responsibility and blame has been lost on the public, which has given much credence to the idea that illness is deserved. A woman diagnosed with breast cancer said, "I couldn't allow myself to be angry at God. But I could allow anger directed at myself. For at some level, due to some imperfection in my character, I thought I had given myself cancer" (Dine, 1982, p. 51). By speaking in the past tense, she appears to indicate that she has reconsidered her conclusion.

But to some, illness, when it occurs, seems to have been the inevitable consequence of past behavior, and not only "bad" behavior. Fritz Zorn (1982) spent the last months of his life writing a book detailing his beliefs about the causes of his illness:

I feel my behavior conformed very well to the rules of society and the rules of cancer. I have been unhappy all my life, but since my good breeding told me it was "not nice" to complain about unhappiness, I never said a word about it. In the world I lived in, tradition demanded that I not create a disturbance or call attention to myself, no matter what the cost to me. I knew that I had to be correct and to conform; above all, I had to be normal. But normality as I understood it meant that I shouldn't tell the truth but should be polite instead. I was a good boy all my life, and that's why I got cancer. That's the way it should be. Anybody who is a good boy all his life deserves to get cancer. It's a just punishment for all that goodness. (p. 121)

This is a shocking confession, and I have no doubt that many holists would want to disavow any association with Zorn's words because they represent the holistic concept taken to its most extreme. The holists must be held accountable when the public picks up one of their statements and articulates the unspoken assumption. When they say, "You are responsible for your health," the public supplies the parenthetical "and your illness is your own damned fault." The holists will protest that this is not what they meant, that the public has distorted their original message. The message has not been distorted; it has simply been carried to its logical conclusion, something perhaps the holists did not think to do. We cannot take seriously the argument that responsibility need not entail blame. Guilt is the natural response of people who perceive they have failed to meet their responsibilities.

And what of the person who has tried to maintain his health and failed? I am always impressed by the anger of the "healthist" who falls ill. On more than one occasion, I have listened to a middle-aged man recite from his hospital bed the litany of things that he did (run, eat a spartan diet) and didn't do (smoke, drink, expose himself to stress) to prevent the heart attack he had just experienced. He expresses rage and frustration at the unfairness of his situation, perhaps some regret at having driven and deprived himself for naught, and nearly always, even in his anger, some guilt that perhaps he hadn't done enough, or done it soon enough.

These people may never have heard of holism, but their anger, frustration, and guilt are a direct consequence of the movement's slogan "You are responsible for your own health."

Illness As Opportunity

Most holists would agree that, if you are going to become sick, you may as well learn something from it. They say that, because illness is often a choice we make, whether consciously or unconsciously, we can gain insight into the reasons for that choice and use it as an opportunity for learning and personal growth. Holists believe that our health choices are fraught with meaning. That is, we do not simply choose to take care of or neglect our health; we do so for a reason. It is imagined that the "meaning" of illness can be revealed through an examination of our health choices. Much confidence is placed in the value of introspection. The ill are encouraged to search their souls honestly for the root causes of their illness.

How very surprising it is to discover that, regardless of the nature or seriousness of the illness, the reason for it is nearly always the same: to allow the individual to meet unfulfilled psychological needs, most often dependency needs. It seems that illness allows us to avoid painful aspects of our lives while enjoying the emotional support that we have been unable to ask for when we are well:

What would it be like to arrive at a place where you could ask for the strokes you need, *when* you need them? Suppose you start viewing your own illness as a need for strokes in some broader context of your life? Imagine the many lessons you would learn, and the growth you could achieve, if you used the experience of disease as an opportunity to reevaluate your lifestyle and environment. What answers might surface if you posed yourself the question "Why do I need this problem at this time?" (Ryan and Travis, 1981, pp. 18 and 21)

Thus, illness is judged to be a maladaptive way of meeting needs and solving problems. It is an opportunity only insofar as sick persons are able to recognize this, discover the nature of their own unmet needs, and invent more constructive ways of fulfilling them. Illness may be an opportunity for patients, but it is equally an opportunity for holists to instruct, patronize, and scold. Their superior understanding allows them special insight into the *real* meaning of their clients' diseases, which they condescend to share with the patient, who mistakenly believe the illness was caused by a virus. In addition, the holist is usually able to prescribe a way to circumvent illness in the future. The Simontons inform their readers that "cancer is a high price to pay to solve problems that could be solved instead by altering your rules so that you give yourself permission to pay attention to your needs" (1980, p. 108).

It is in keeping with the holistic bias toward psychological etiologies that the ultimate meaning of illness is interpreted in psychological terms. In spite of the movement's professed interest in social and environmental influences, little attention is given to these as either cause or meaning. Could my emphysema mean, simply, that I am involuntarily exposed to industrial pollutants? (Holists like to point out that, though many people are exposed to a particular threat, only a few become ill. A psychological vulnerability is posited to explain this. However, such vulnerability has never been demonstrated to be either a necessary or sufficient cause of *any* physical illness.) Greater social than psychological significance can be found in the numbers of children from poor families who suffer from lead poisoning. Even stress—that nemesis of holistic health—may be of social rather than psychic origin and hence not readily controlled by the individual. When Shealy (1979) claims that "most people are born with good health and lose it through poor habits and stressful lifestyles" (p. 1294), we have to ask if he views starvation as a poor habit, or poverty as a life-style.

Nor do holists search for a larger meaning in suffering that would allow them to transcend personal or social considerations. Viktor Frankl (1963) believes that illness can teach us to value that which is truly important in our lives and that suffering may provide us with the opportunity to act with dignity and responsibility. He believes that our lives, and therefore events in our lives such as suffering, hold a meaning larger than ourselves that may relate to personal relationships or to ultimate values. Some, like Job, seek the meaning of affliction in their relationship with God. The holistic understanding of the meaning of illness is smaller, more personal, less willing to admit that forces may exist that are larger than or beyond the control of the individual. There is a distinct reluctance to admit that sometimes disease and suffering do not have a readily identifiable meaning. An essentially a-religious movement (in spite of the inevitable reference to the "spiritual" component), holism, unable to tolerate the possibility of randomness, blames the individual rather than God.

Sontag claims that "nothing is more punitive than to give a disease a meaning—that meaning being invariably a moralistic one" (p. 57). I would argue that the kind of meaning Frankl describes is not punitive, but uplifting, supportive of the sufferer. The meaning sought by the holists, however, can indeed be punitive. Diamant (1982) observes that, though illness may provide people with the opportunity to learn something about themselves, the gain is not necessarily worth the price:

> Some patients, and the practitioners observing them, re-port life-changing insights into family relationships and self-destructive patterns, insights that may contribute to a much-improved quality of life, for however long they survive. . . . To suggest that such insights and growth can make up for the suffering of cancer would be cruel and stupid. But to deny the impact of such hard-won understanding would be equally arrogant. (p. 8)

If illness is an opportunity, then death is, in the sales cliché, the opportunity of a lifetime. It is not the end of growth, but another occasion for growth. It is "increasingly being recognized as an important, albeit final, opportunity for growth and transformation" (Lappé, 1979, p. 478). Again, the desperate need for personal control is evident. Although many seek meaning in death, and a "meaningless" death is considered particularly painful, the holist desires not only to understand the event but to control it.

Summary

As the unit of interest in the holistic scheme, individuals are made to carry a heavy burden. They must do what no one else has been entirely successful in doing: prevent illness from occurring. As Keller (1981) notes, "Health would seem to be quite an obligation!" (p. 50). If it is to be possible for the individual to prevent illness, three requirements will have to be met. First, causality must be established; second, rules of behavior enabling the person to avoid the known causes must be fixed; and, third, it must be possible for the person to carry out the prescribed preventive measures. To date, these requirements have not been met for many illnesses. It is therefore premature to assign complete responsibility to the individual.

That the holists have done so is partly the result of naiveté. They have shown too much enthusiasm for anecdotal evidence, too much readiness to accept those partial truths that support their views. They extrapolate from the evidence to presently insupportable conclusions. Their worst excess is in suggesting that emotions cause or can cure illness. Indirectly, a case could be made that anxiety causes me to smoke, thereby contributing to bronchitis, or that anxiety over the possible consequences could lead me to stop smoking. This is not to say, as the holists do, that emotions can be the direct cause of illness.

Until we know more about the relationship between illness and emotion, such a suggestion is highly irresponsible, leading, as has been discussed, to much anguish on the part of the person who has failed to stay well. It has been noted that stress, itself believed to contribute to illness, is actually increased by the emphasis on personal accountability.

There may be reasons other than naiveté that preventive measures used by the individual are so highly regarded. It is arguably easier to treat those who are not ill. The therapist can claim a victory even when nothing

happens, pointing happily to the client who did not fall
ill. Of course, statistical evidence is good that certain
preventive measures are effective. For example, populations whose water supply is fluoridated suffer from
fewer dental caries. Some holistic therapies will un-
doubtedly be shown to be of value too, but the efficacy
of much of the holistic armamentarium remains to be
proved. In the meantime, the fact that a holist remains
well does not constitute evidence that special techniques
have thwarted an illness that would otherwise have developed.

The dogma of personal responsibility has also altered
the manner in which manifest disease is handled. The
focus is shifted from practitioner to client, who is an-
swerable for the results of therapy, thus removing a significant burden from the practitioner. Conventional
health-care providers are well aware that, when treatment fails, the practitioner may stand accused of incom-
petence or even fraud. The holistic practitioner need not
be concerned with this because failure to respond to
treatment is viewed as the fault of the patient, from
whom all healing comes. The practitioner is merely a
kind of coach who provides encouragement for the *vis
medicatrix naturae*. Naturally, patients who stubbornly refuse to cooperate will not get better. The therapist cannot
be held liable and may disavow responsibility for the
outcome with some hostility. Monaco (1978) warns:
"Don't expect me to assume full responsibility for YOUR
health" (p. 10).

Too much emphasis has been placed in the movement
on what individuals can and should do for themselves
and too little on what they can expect from professional
care providers. There is also too little recognition of the
limits of personal endeavor and will power. Expectations
have been created that cannot be met and, when they

are not, much unhappiness results. It would be a responsible act for the holists to acknowledge their contribution to this situation and help educate the public in a more realistic understanding of the cause and cure of illness.

5

Society, Community, and Values

Many reasons have been given to explain the sudden appearance and continuing popularity of the holistic health movement, most of them having to do with the failings of allopathic medicine. It is certainly true that many who turn to holism are seeking an alternative to the expensive, highly technical (and sometimes impersonal and ineffective) care provided by conventional practitioners. But allopathic medicine has been the dominant force in health care since early in this century. It has always had its faults and its critics, and alternatives such as chiropractic and homeopathy have always been available. Dissatisfaction with conventional care, then, does not fully explain the growth of the new movement.

What forces have encouraged the advance of holistic health and its particular value system at this time and in this place? I believe the answer can be found in the social changes immediately preceding and accompanying the establishment of the movement. It would be too simple an explanation to say that middle-class Americans simply became more aware of and concerned about personal health. Although the emphasis in holism is on the individual, social factors stronger than a common valuing of health are stimulating the phenomenon of the health-anxious American. As Ivan Illich says, "To a large extent culture and health coincide" (1977a, p. 122).

Holistic health, emphasizing as it does individual initiative, may be a very American sort of idea. Lipowski (1981), discussing the holistic approach in psychiatry, claims that "it is an approach that could only flourish in a pluralistic, open, and democratic society, since it is the product of the liberal mind" (p. 895). And Mattson (1982) notes that the holistic belief in self-responsibility "would be unthinkable in other cultural contexts. It could be applicable only in a highly individualistic, 'I-centered' culture where each person is encouraged to find his or her own lifestyle among many choices" (p. 41). This chapter will argue that interest in holistic health is one response to the rapid social change of the past two decades and that its value system both reflects and contributes to the prevailing values of the times.

Loss of Community

Many people today have an uncomfortable sense that their lives are becoming more complicated, less subject to their control. They may feel that their place in the world has become less significant. At work they find they can be replaced by a machine or by any of a number of other persons. Their role at home may disappear through divorce or disinterest on the part of family members. They see little chance that they can influence events in the community or the nation. In short, they feel diminished.

Morgan (1968) argues that what is occurring is nothing less than the dissolution of the person. According to him, many forces are conspiring to threaten our integrity as whole human beings. One is the replacement of the conception of man as at least partly self-determining with one that regards him as merely reacting to forces outside his control. Along with this has arisen a bias toward a reductionistic interpretation of distinctively human characteristics, such as creativity, religious feeling, and the formation of values. Morgan believes too, that the expression of feelings is being discouraged because emotional life is devalued. Feelings are suspect; they are not to be considered in decisions because they are "subjective"—or worse, "irrational." Reasoning itself is limited to scientific rationality—there is no wisdom, only knowledge:

> Human activities are atomized; none is considered in the light of what it does to the remainder of life. The human self is fragmented into faculties and interests that ignore or suppress each other. Action is separated from moral sense, reason is split from feeling, life is deprived of understanding, and understanding is divorced from life. (p. 76)

The stripped-down model of the person cannot seek support for his remaining personhood in the community. He is too small to be noticed and too weak to be effective:

> In all parts of our life we are constantly confronted with things whose vast scale far exceeds the individual's size and powers. We rarely live or work in a community in which our presence counts and is felt, and in which the circumstances we must confront are of human dimensions. The enormity of all organizations and institutions, the hugeness of the political apparatus, the appalling rush of events, and the unthinkable powers of extermi-

nation that constantly hover over us, all threaten to crush us into impotence. (p. 66)

Morgan makes a powerful argument that human wholeness cannot be achieved when "we are not given the conditions necessary to define and shape ourselves as persons" (p. 66). His description of wholeness is more compelling than the simpler mind-body-spirit unity model of the holists, but the dissolution he speaks of is surely one of the prime elements in the growth of the movement, more significant perhaps than the dissatisfaction with conventional medicine. We *do* have a need to realize ourselves fully in the context of a group, a family, and a community that cares. The holistic health movement is a response to the frustration of that need.

Before health emerged as an important theme in the counterculture where the holistic movement has roots, strong emphasis was placed on the wholeness and healing power of community. At the height of the counterculture, Passmore (1970) wrote that young people were attracted to "the mystical idea of 'unity.' The young generation responds, so we are told, 'to the sense and sound of friendship and community, to the exultation they feel when thousands of people link hands and sing *We shall overcome*' " (p. 309). This motif is echoed, unchanged by a holist who says: "Healing is circle-dancing and singing to 'Rocking on the Water' at [a] . . . concert with six of your closest friends . . . ending with a deep, satisfying hug" (Smith, D., 1982, p. 21).

Passmore claims that the search for total unity is within the perfectibilist tradition:

The young are rebelling, in part, against the atomistic tendencies of modern society. But they have reacted, in

the manner only too typical of human beings, by revert-
ing to the old perfectibilist, and in the end tyrannical,
ideal of a total unity rather than the admittedly more
complex ideal of a plurality of intersecting communities.
(p. 310)

Passmore contends that, because total unity, harmony,
and order are beyond the reach of humans, systems that
demand them are threats to human diversity, and hence
are de-humanizing. Holistic health seeks unity not
among peoples, but within the person. To the extent that
it suppresses diversity among individuals by labeling deviation from a pre-established ideal "sick," it too is de-
humanizing.

Although the counterculture focused on the value of
the community, the seeds of individualism that would
later blossom in the holistic health movement were already present. Reich asserts: "Consciousness III starts
with self. In contrast to Consciousness II, which accepts
society, the public interest, and institutions as the primary reality, III declares that the individual self is the
only true reality" (1970, p. 225). He then offers the pre-
dictable disclaimer that to be concerned with self is not
necessarily to be selfish.

It is true that the counterculture was often characterized by a generosity toward others. But, perhaps because
the need for community remained unfulfilled, the focus
began to shift from the group to the person. Shaffer
(1978) observes that, by 1970, interest in encounter
groups was being replaced by meditation. Now, in the
late 1980s, the shift is complete and the unit of interest
is the individual. Of particular concern to the holist is
personal health. But because, as we have seen, that en-
compasses just about everything, the enormity of self-
interest is staggering.

People are encouraged to examine each aspect of their lives for its contribution to health. After all, we are told, it is our responsibility. Thus, we see people paying increasing attention to themselves in the name of good health. Encouraged by their physicians, teachers, and ministers as well as by advertising and insurance companies, they gain a heightened awareness of themselves. What in the past might have been dismissed as self-absorption is now sanctioned as "health behavior."

But this is not occurring in a vacuum. I believe that our concern with personal health is a reflection of changes occurring in American society that have created the narcissistic culture described by Lasch (1979). As he points out, "Social change manifests itself inwardly as well as outwardly, in changing perceptions, habits of mind, unconscious associations" (p. 355). The narcissistic culture has created an atmosphere in which self-preoccupation is not only tolerated, but is the norm.

The resulting narcissistic personality type manifests narcissism partly in intense involvement in matters concerning well-being. A system, or therapeutic, to use Rieff's (1968) term, has been created in which any behavior or attitude that contributes to health is seen as positive and desirable. Those that do not foster health are without value, and those that may harm health are unacceptable. In this framework, the concepts of good and bad, moral and immoral are simply irrelevant.

Health and Holism in a Narcissistic Society

"Culture," says Rieff, "is another name for a design of motives directing the self outward, toward those communal purposes in which alone the self can be realized and satisfied" (p. 4). He goes on to argue forcefully that we are moving inexorably away from the communal purposes that defined our lives in the past and toward a future in which individuals will be increasingly isolated, and communal purposes but a quaint relic from the past. As social endeavors lose their importance, individual aspirations and efforts will gain dominance. "The new center, which can be held even as communities disintegrate, is the self" (p. 5). Institutions that formerly laid claim to our loyalties now falter and fade. Religion, as Rieff points out, is no longer the organizing principle for as many lives as it was once. Its authority is diminished. Churches sometimes offer more social activities than worship services.

Other institutions that might have lured us away from ourselves are changing or failing. The community loses its power to compel selfless behavior in the interest of the group. The governing of our larger, national community becomes more difficult as the ideal of patriotism is lost, replaced by single-interest groups. Even the family fractures into individuals needing their own "space" and seeking private paths to "personal growth."

Lasch suggests that the phenomenon of the individual rising Phoenix-like from the ashes of our institutions is the end-product of a culture that has long fostered personal achievement through competition:

> . . . the culture of competitive individualism, which in its decadence has carried the logic of individualism to the extreme of a war of all against all, the pursuit of happiness to the dead end of a narcissistic preoccupation with the self. (p. 21)

The self, then, replaces community. But, if Rieff is correct, if the self can only be realized and satisfied by commitment to communal purpose, what will nurture it once the social institutions which have served that purpose in the past have withered? Nothing has appeared on the horizon showing promise of being able to replace that which is being destroyed.

The individual, shorn of the meaning a community can provide, is seeking fulfillment, not by building new communities and relationships, but by using various resources for personal nourishment, enhancement, and celebration. Ingenious ways of doing so have been found. Selection can be made from an astonishing variety of books, courses, activities, and regimens designed only for personal nurture and self-preoccupation. One need only look at the titles available in the health section of a bookstore to gain some idea of the breadth of this type of self-interest:

Overcoming the Fear of Success
How to Flatten Your Stomach
Success Through a Positive Mental Attitude
Maximum Personal Energy
Psychological War on Fat
Growing New Hair!
Creative Dreaming
How to Look Ten Years Younger
Natural Breast Enlargement

We are becoming a nation of therapeutics, to use Rieff's term. They assign value to ideas and behaviors only to the extent that they "work" for themselves. They are indifferent to the notion of community values and to the larger issues of morality. Indeed, they are indifferent to anything not directly related to themselves. Rieff asks: "What would suit the therapeutic ideal better than the prevalent American piety toward the self? This self, improved, is the ultimate concern of modern culture" (p. 62).

The improved self is rapidly being reinterpreted as the healthy self. Because the therapeutics' interest in themselves is unlimited, they eagerly endorse the more grandiose definitions of health. Not for them is the idea of health as absence of disease. They seek to include every facet of themselves in the definition. Their fascination with themselves is such that they cannot imagine themselves as healthy if some part is functioning less than adequately. They will inevitably, therefore, be attracted to holistic formulations of health.

The failure of our society to provide us with institutions and principles that compel our allegiance has created an atmosphere in which therapeutic (holistic) man flourishes. Man pays homage to himself. But the loss of community leaves him anxious because he is unable to fill the void left by the loss. Left with only himself, the self takes on an exaggerated importance. The person who abandons—or is abandoned by—God, community, and family clings to what is left: himself. He must seek every means to protect that self for it is all-important; there is nothing else. Because the self is all, each part of the self has importance. The therapeutic is so enamored of each facet of himself that he frantically seeks to nurture each part. The popular press and lay public have picked up the buzz word. One can attend classes on holistic child-rearing, read about holistic architectural design, and practice a holistic approach to exercise by meditating while jogging.

The desperation of narcissists has contributed to the growing popularity of holism. What could be of more interest to them than their "whole" selves? They reject the more modest definitions of holism as not doing justice to themselves. It is not enough, they argue, to claim a relationship between mind and body because the parts are inseparable in the function of the whole. One could not talk about the mind affecting the body or vice versa because mind and body are one; regarded in isolation, they become meaningless artifacts. Further, and most importantly for narcissists, the integrated mind-body model fails to account for their dazzling complexity. They see mind-body as a naive reduction that neglects much of what contributes to their wholeness. They are more than mind and body. Their wholeness depends on their spirit, intellect, emotions, sexuality, social relations, fitness, and environment as well.

Narcissists, in their self-concern, cannot feel well unless each area is attended to. Holism represents for them a justification of their narcissism. They are able to fret about themselves incessantly with the full support and encouragement of peers and professionals in the name of health. Because they are concerned about more than their physical well-being, they begin to subsume all kinds of activities under the heading of "health-promoting behaviors." Matters that once might have been considered business, legal, or social concerns are now labeled health concerns.

Lasch explains how American progressivism has contributed to this trend.

> It has rejected the liberal conception of man . . . and has installed in its place a therapeutic conception. . . . It has rejected the stereotype of economic man and has attempted to bring the "whole man" under social control. Instead of regulating the conditions of work alone, it now regulates private life as well, organizing leisure time on scientific principles of social and personal hygiene. It has

exposed the innermost secrets of the psyche to medical
scrutiny and has thus encouraged habits of anxious self-
scrutiny. (pp. 378–379)

Thus do both the individual and society foster narcissism
in the name of health. Holism as a manifestation of narcissism has developed so insidiously that few recognize
the relationship. The exception is the current fitness
craze and the attendant vanity. It has been noted that
many people exercise not for good health but for good
looks (Reed, 1981).

Holistic health passes itself off as a system that offers
a superior understanding of human nature. Moreover,
it holds out the promise of a better life to those who
accept its dogma. In this sense, it can be seen as an ersatz
religion. But, unlike religious traditions that seek meaning in sources outside the self, holism has no transcendent quality. Its disciples look inward, seeking salvation
by their own hands. This pseudo-religious quality has
an element of self-righteousness. We are told that we
have not only a right, but an *obligation* to care for ourselves. Those not in the fold are pitied, even scorned,
for their failure to live a healthy life as defined by the
holists. The converted take smug satisfaction in the in-
ordinate care with which they perform the prescribed
rituals.

Duhl (1979) notes that "in some ways, hospitals and
the medical establishment have replaced cathedrals and
the Church as the focal points of attention in a society
that at one time hoped and dreamed that the Church
could provide answers to questions regarding the totality
of existence. The medieval church, as strong as it was,
proved unable to do this and we as physicians are—or
should be—too wise to claim that we are capable of dealing with such broad issues" (p. 473). Holistic physicians,

though holding no such reservations, are no better qualified to address such issues. Their movement evolved in response to, but could not meet, the need for community and meaning. The failure was inevitable. The philosophy of the movement was always too weak to meet that challenge. Instead, it shrank away, narrowed its concern to the individual, and thus helped to compound the original problems of isolation and meaninglessness.

Loss of Values

Along with the loss of community, we are experiencing a loss of values. Mom, church, and apple pie no longer symbolize prevailing American values. People seldom affirm absolute commitment to anything significant. Behaviors such as monogamy, civic ideals such as patriotism, and individual characteristics such as integrity are regarded now as personal proclivities. Morgan (1968) attributes the disappearance of compelling values largely to the increasing belief that they are entirely subjective and merely represent the likes and dislikes or desires of the individual. He notes that the anthropological doctrine of cultural relativism has contributed to the belief that no one behavior or ideal is better than another, just different. This relativistic stance is also an inheritance from the counterculture's "do-your-own-thing" philosophy.

A complete absence of values, however, can hardly be tolerated by most of us. It does not bring freedom, as is often hoped, but chaos and loss of direction. It is disorienting rather than exhilarating. Some values are discarded because they make us morally uncomfortable when we betray them. Others are rightly abandoned as false or unnecessarily provincial and restricting. Something must take their place. Morgan contends that we will search wildly for replacements:

> Without values there is emptiness, boredom, and desperation. Without values individuals and society disintegrate. Or terror arises, and men frantically erect new things to function as values; they seize upon anything—idols, isms, slogans, or lies—to give purpose to their lives; and they pursue these pseudo values with fanatic and often bloody single-mindedness. (p. 26)

Holism is just such an "ism" for many. Its adherents are very likely to be those for whom other values have been lost. Mattson (1982), in a survey of sixteen holistic healers, asked what factors led them to their decisions to pursue that role. Among the factors identified were marriage problems (63%), apostasy (63%), and identity crisis (81%) (p. 108). The rush toward holism is a rush away from lost values of home, faith, and self-worth in the urgent hope that replacements can be found. The person who has an "identity crisis" may assume a new role as a holist, an expert, perhaps even a healer. Someone experiencing troubled personal relationships may seek new ones within the brotherhood of holism, where most vagaries (except poor health habits) are met with "unconditional positive regard." Lost religious faith is replaced with faith in holistic doctrine and ritual.

This is why the slogans of the movement have achieved such power. They are a form of creed, distilled statements of belief that can be chanted in moments of crisis. Holists who are feeling assaulted by events seemingly beyond their control can take comfort in remembering that at least "You are responsible for your own health." And, if the forces of conventional medicine mount a challenge to holism, the former can be attacked and the latter affirmed in the same breath, with the shout: "Health is more than the absence of disease!"

The slogans are statements of values, or rather are statements about *the* value selected by the holists: good health. In a world that is complex and sometimes threatening, it is difficult to know which values are worth holding, difficult to reconcile competing values, still more difficult to be worthy of the values we do choose. How much simpler to select only one, elevate it above all others, and disregard the rest: one value—health—which literally *embodies* the ideals of simplicity, order, harmony, and unity. It is no wonder that a movement which offers these draws converts from older value systems that are more complicated and demanding.

Pseudo-Values and Silent Values

According to Dubos (1980), "Good health implies an individual's success in functioning within his particular set of values, and as such is extremely relative" (p. 547). But what if the particular set of values is bad? It would not seem reasonable to suggest that personal health is a bad value, but it becomes a bad or at least a distorted value if it is the only one. Isolating health or any other value from all others turns it from a genuine into a pseudo-value. As Morgan has explained:

> Choice and commitment imply valuation, and valuation, like freedom, is linked with wholeness, for when any part of life is segregated from the rest, assessment of that part becomes impossible. Only if one part is balanced with other parts—only if it is seen in concrete context, and if all parts of the world and all parts of the self involved in

a particular occasion are acknowledged and reconciled—
can there be true valuation. Otherwise values become
pseudo values—interests, methods, or goals isolated
from all else, set up as values, and blindly affirmed. (p.
326)

Health has been extracted from its context and ac-
corded the status of a super-value. It is not seen as something that contributes to our ability to live well and to
honor other values. It is considered valuable in and of
itself. Vargiu and Remen ask: "Is human health indeed
only an end in itself, or is it actually a means toward a
greater goal? . . . Is the current drive towards physical
health as the ultimate goal and defense against death at
any cost really the best and most satisfying way to live?"
(1979, p. 472). Too many holists think so. LeShan (1982)
describes the chronic "get-in-shapers" who pursue
health via nutrition, exercise, or meditation. "If you ask
them what they are getting in shape *for*—how they plan
to use the work in one domain to increase the artistic
pattern and expression of their whole lives—they look
at you blankly. The means has replaced the end" (p. 127).
Living by any pseudo-value (which health is when it is
isolated) cannot be satisfying because it causes us to ignore other aspects of ourselves and the world. Ironically,
the exclusive attention holists give to health is itself reductionistic and contributes to the dissolution of wholeness.

Still, the assumption that personal health is the highest
value is not seriously questioned. Enthusiasts have succeeded in disguising the underlying narcissism of this
assumption by presenting health as an obligation rather
than a blessing. It is something we are responsible for.
The "shoulds" and "musts" rain down hard and heavy.
We should stop smoking, relax more, foster outside in-

terests. Holists grandly instruct us that we have the power to be well and the duty to use it. They do not hesitate to insist that each of us devote our energies to the task of achieving the highest possible level of wellness. None are excused from this obligation. Woe to the sedentary souls who prefer reading in an armchair to physical activity. They will soon be reminded that both body and mind need exercise. Such is the power of holistic thought in our culture that it may not even occur to them that they may be as healthy as more well-rounded types.

Holists have a way of flattening the differences between people. All must conform to the ideal. So much for athletes who are no great thinkers, or social activists who neglect their diets while doing community organizing. Ernest Becker (1968) suggests that "the free, tense individual may want to sacrifice his health to higher symbolic values" (p. 298). But no real consideration is given to the possibility that other values may be equally or more important than health. It has become such a struggle for holists to achieve health that they neglect to question whether the struggle is worth the prize.

Hidden behind the super-value is a subset of unspoken, silent values—assumptions really. Holists themselves are unlikely to be aware of them and, if confronted with them, would deny holding them, for they expose a darker, less tolerant, and more vulnerable aspect of the movement. One is that wholeness is necessary to health (and therefore to happiness and a worthwhile life). This in itself might be acknowledged by those in the movement, but it prompts a question: What are the consequences for the person who is structurally or functionally less than whole? A dozen examples come to mind: people who are blind, who have had amputations, who are paralyzed, who are retarded. Being less than whole, can they ever be healthy? Can they realize a meaningful life? Indeed, are they even fully human?

One of the difficulties here is the previously mentioned failure to provide an adequate description of human wholeness. Zaner (1981) states: "A theory of actively constituted and experienced bodily integrity or wholeness is necessary to medicine and biomedical science" (p. 32). That others have experienced difficulty in this effort does not excuse the holists, whose entire movement is based on the notion of wholeness. Lacking such a theory, they would deny that persons having some kind of deficit are necessarily less than healthy or whole and claim that those people could achieve a kind of functional wholeness within their limits. Perhaps man is not such an indivisible unity as was previously imagined, but has a unified core of self and some nonessential parts as well, which may be disposed of without violating the whole. Could it be that Descartes was correct in observing: "When a foot, an arm, or any other part is cut off, I am conscious that nothing has been taken from the mind"?

But this is the kind of back-pedaling holists engage in when one of their tenets is revealed to have less than admirable consequences. I suspect that their original statements about the relationship between health, wholeness, and personhood actually reveal their true feelings quite clearly. How many holists could sustain the loss of a part or function without experiencing themselves as terribly mutilated? As Cassel (1982) notes, "If suffering occurs when there is a threat to one's integrity or a loss of a part of a person, then suffering will continue if the person cannot be made whole again" (p. 644).

Those who worship wholeness create suffering for those whose wholeness is broken. An attempt is made to avoid accepting responsibility for this outcome by supposing that wholeness can be maintained indefinitely, if only the prescribed way of life is followed. Holists are usually careful to say that illness may sometimes occur, that some accidents are unavoidable, that, as one pointed out, the mortality rate is still 100 percent. Nevertheless, there is an underlying belief (or hope) that disease, infirmity, aging, and death are not inevitable. This is not articulated, but is another silent assumption.

Holists are generally well-educated people who do not wish to invite ridicule and who, on some level, realize the impossibility of avoiding all suffering. Yet, their literature reveals an inchoate hope that one *might*, by dint of wanting enough and working enough, make it so. There is a sense that *if only*—what? If only I take the right minerals in the right combination. If only I breathe correctly, relax completely, eliminate enough toxins . . . then surely I will be well.

This sense of "if only" may account for the ever-increasing number of therapies. When the chosen treatment fails to provide perfect health, it is not because the goal is unattainable but because the therapy is incorrect for that person at that time. If not iridology or herbology, then perhaps some other "ology" will be the answer. The search must continue because holists find the alternative too terrifying. They cannot accept that they will be ill, age, and die. Underneath the cheerful countenance and the expressions of confidence in their ability to control their health lies tremendous anxiety, even desperation. Only their denial prevents them from fully experiencing it.

When holists encounter a situation in which they are forced to acknowledge the reality of suffering, in an apparent about-face, they proclaim that disease holds important meanings for us and that illness and even death provide us with grand opportunities for learning and growing. But this glorification of suffering is also a form of denial that permits holists to believe that somehow they can escape the human condition. A psychiatrist might call this a reaction formation, but perhaps it is more a narcissistic response on the part of those who believe that, for them, the usual rules will be suspended. They do not understand, as does Morgan, that "there is no final perfection to be reached" (p. 330). Human frailty and mortality belong to each of us.

Summary

The holistic health movement is not only an inadequate but also a distorted response to the problems of loss of community and loss of values—one that magnifies the problems it intends to correct. In a narcissistic culture, personal well-being looms large. Social institutions that once absorbed our energy and commanded our loyalty fail as we desert them. Turning away from communal concerns, we turn inward toward the self. As the self-absorption of individuals increases, they begin to interpret all experience in terms of their own welfare. In this they are supported by a society that is increasingly structured to nurture individual rather than group aspirations. As the self-concern of narcissists grows, their concept of health becomes more grandiose. When all of life is seen as affecting health, the transformation from narcissist to holist is complete.

Holists have not adequately explored the possibility that there may be more worthy values than personal health. Certainly other values have prevailed in the past. The ideals of service to community, sacrifice of self for family, and devotion to a religious life were admired, if not always practiced. Self-involvement was not. The holists have neatly turned things upside down, and it is a tribute to their sleight-of-hand that no one has noticed. Self-sacrifice becomes sacrifice in the service of the self. This is the consequence of a culture that encourages unlimited self-interest and is structured to provide for the smallest need of the individual at the expense of communal purposes.

6

Holism and the Health Professions

The conventional health professions came late to the holistic revolution. A fantastic variety of unlicensed healers
was already practicing before traditional providers took
any serious note of them. The holists were frequently
dismissed out of hand as charlatans: useless or dangerous or both. This response was due, in part, to the fact
that many were at pains to represent themselves as exotic, and often advertised their lack of formal training as
an advantage. In a widely read book on holistic health,
one of the authors was described as follows:

> [She] has served as an administrator with the Berkeley
> Holistic Health Center. A masseuse, flamenco dancer, and
> metaphysical practitioner, she is currently complet-
> ing a program to become a professional prayer therapist
> through the Teaching of the Inner Christ, a nonsectarian
> metaphysical fellowship. (Berkeley Holistic Health Cen-
> ter, 1978, p. 480)

Licensed providers found it easy to scorn or ignore
those kinds of credentials, and, during its early years, the
holistic health movement increased remarkably in size
and influence. Whether this occurred in spite of or be-

cause of the lack of attention from conventional providers is not clear. Nevertheless, when they did begin to take note of the movement, they found it flourishing.

Conventional Health Care Turns toward Holism

By the late 1970s, many references to holism began to appear in the health-care literature. Interest increased and remains high today, as evidenced by the large number of books and articles devoted to the topic. Perhaps equally significant are the many passing references to holism in papers concerned with other subjects. We must wonder why so many conventional practitioners have abandoned their earlier indifference or hostility. To be sure, not all have embraced holism; some vociferously reject its tenets and practices. But it has engaged the interest of enough practitioners to have become an important theme.

Some of the growing fascination with holism was a response to criticisms framed by newly articulate "consumers" of health-care services. Kestenbaum (1982) observes that, "at the same time that health and the body became a secure part of the cultural consciousness, the professions responsible for the health needs of the country entered the cultural consciousness. One awakening was appreciative and positive, the other critical and negative" (pp. 3–4). In responding to the grievances of consumers, many conventional practitioners were influenced by the "appreciative and positive" aspects of holism.

Still, other alternatives were available. Conventional practitioners might have chosen to address costs of treatment, allocation of resources, or the efficacy of highly technical therapies—all of which were objects of censure (Berliner and Salmon, 1980). Instead, they chose to embrace holism, which emphasized the relational aspects of health care. What was the reason behind the choice? Or, in the harsh terms of one critic, "Why this particular quackery at this particular time?" (Edlund, 1983, p. 800).

Clearly, the original holists and the newly holistic conventional providers have recognized a need to attend to the deteriorating relationship between provider and client. Dubos (1979a) has argued that what he terms "fringe medicine" owes its popularity "to the failure of the present biomedical sciences to satisfy some large human needs" (p. 211). Technical competence, even virtuosity, is not enough if delivered by an arrogant or indifferent practitioner who is not sensitive to the experience of the patient. Finding that they had "large human needs" that were not being met, some patients drifted towards holism, to be followed later by those practitioners who recognized the problem and thought they saw an answer in the movement. Pellegrino (1982) asserts that, though physicians may emphasize technical competence, patients seek "compassionate help with the experience of illness" (p. 160). This, he maintains, constitutes a gap between the two parties' understanding of the healing relationship:

> This gap promises to widen as specialism increases and the demands of competence become more urgent. The wider it becomes the more remote is a genuine healing relationship grounded in the experience of illness. The stronger, too, will be the urge for patients to seek alternatives to the "medical model." The opposite danger— that of losing the benefits of scientific competence—then presents itself. (pp. 160–161)

As the possibility that patients would seek alternatives became manifest reality, providers became alarmed and, rather than see patients lost to conventional care altogether, sought to change the nature of such care to better meet the need for "compassionate help with the experience of illness." To some extent, they themselves became part of the alternative.

The avant-garde of the movement among professional care givers toward holism was made up of the so-called allied health professionals—those nonphysician, licensed persons who provide health care. Several possibilities present themselves as to why this might be so. First, these professions tend to be of more recent origin than medicine. They may be more open to criticism as they seek to shape their own identity as distinct from medicine. Kestenbaum (1982) notes that criticism from patients prompted those in the allied professions to engage in some self-criticism as well: "Nurses, occupational therapists, physical therapists, and others were relentlessly critical of the medical model. . . . By the end of the seventies it became risky to talk about 'medicine and health care professionals' as if they all shared a common culture" (p. 8). For some, a crucial difference between their profession and that of medicine was the use of a holistic approach.

Second, some groups identified holism as a new term for something that had long been a part of their practice. Nurses, particularly, believed that they represented a long tradition of holistic-type care. Other groups, too, have asserted that, though they may not have articulated it as such, their approach has always been fundamentally holistic.

Finally, it may be that the "allieds" have turned to holism in an attempt to stake out a claim for themselves.

These groups, so often overshadowed and even bullied by the wealthier and more influential medical profession, may see in holism an opportunity to establish themselves as offering a unique kind of health care. They may see themselves, and represent themselves to potential clients, as capable of caring more effectively for the whole person than can the physician, who may be unsuited to this kind of care by virtue of his or her highly specialized education or lack of interest in anything beyond the diseased part.

Medical doctors are now well represented in the ranks of holists. Membership in the American Holistic Medical Association is restricted exclusively to M.D.'s. In general, however, physicians have been slow to join the movement, and their response to it has not been universally positive. Some remain largely ignorant of it; others are outright hostile. As Davies (1979) notes:

> Many physicians have never heard of holistic health care or high-level wellness. It is hard for them to believe that intelligent, well-educated, articulate people can espouse alternatives to the traditional health care system. Once the incredulity wears off, the response usually falls somewhere between balderdash and poppycock. (p. 1357)

A number of physicians have asserted—some with much heat—that the tenets of holism are nothing new, but represent understandings long recognized and used by their profession. Relman (1979) asks if experienced and skillful physicians have not always dealt with patients and not diseases, recognized psychological and social factors in disease, and encouraged patients to be involved in treatment. "Who can quarrel with those insights? . . . If these are the lessons of holistic medicine, they should be welcomed as old friends" (p. 312).

A typical response of those physicians who voice some support for holism is to express approval with reservations. Yahn (1979) suggests that nonphysicians be allowed to practice health care only if they are licensed. Frank (1981) allows that a physician may seriously consider "those aspects of the holistic orientation that do not conflict with his world-view" (p. 227). Those M.D.'s who are more enthusiastic are likely to espouse "integration" or "complementarity." That is, they believe that a holistic perspective is not necessarily inimical to the practice of conventional medicine. They would like to see the two blended to take advantage of the best of each. Finally, some doctors wholeheartedly embrace holism as a superior orientation and would like to see conventional medicine adopt its perspective without reservation.

We should now return to the question posed earlier in this chapter concerning the reasons for the move toward holism among health professionals, and ask more particularly why so many physicians are advocating holism to a greater or lesser degree. It is important to recall that physicians were latecomers, arriving to find other groups already well established and claiming to offer different and even superior services than those available from physicians or physician-controlled agencies. Doctors found that their traditional authority was being undermined and their previously exclusive territory being encroached on by nurses and other health-care providers. Salmon and Berliner (1980) speculate that "holism together with self-care [may] . . . contribute to a further abandonment of established provider institutions" (p. 546). Abandonment by patients will not only diminish the influence of doctors, but will decrease the income they are able to realize as the dominant health-care group. Carlson (1979) cites loss of stature and money as one reason they are unwilling to share responsibility with other health professionals.

It is not insignificant that the threats to the economic security of physicians by the holistic health movement were occurring at a time of rapid expansion of the physician population of the United States (Ginzberg, 1985). Not only were M.D.'s in competition with other professionals, but intraprofessional competition was increasing as well. Some physicians, seeing an opportunity, began looking more kindly at the interest in holistic health. As the definition of health expanded, the possibilities for treatment broadened, and some physicians began offering therapy for stress, for example. As physicians go, so go physician-dominated institutions, and hospitals began to offer nontraditional services, such as behavioral medicine and sports medicine. In the mid-1980s, federal cost-containment measures aimed at controlling Medicare expenditures caused hospitals to rely even more heavily on income from nontraditional services that do not rely on third-party reimbursement. Thus, economic considerations made holistic therapies more attractive to physicians.

Another challenge to the dominance of M.D.'s was the claim of some holistic providers that they offered care in a more sensitive manner and were more attuned to the patient's experience. Nurses and others suggested that they could offer viable alternatives to an exclusively physician-controlled system. The threat to the medical establishment was clear. Doctors who were ostensibly concerned with warning the public about the dangers of poorly trained practitioners revealed, perhaps, another consideration in their rather crude use of the term "piece of the action":

> In the future, of course, we will see holistic "factories" and a further proliferation of minimally trained para-professionals who want a piece of the action. (Lemkin, 1980, p. 363)

> But society should be aware of the charlatans who advertise themselves as holistic healers, yet who are without any special qualifications. We can see a full complement of colorful characters . . . Chinese herbalists, psychiatric healers, Indian shamans and some medical doctors all vying for a "piece of the action." (Todd, 1979, p. 465)

The physicians themselves, of course, have reason to fear losing their own "piece of the action." In response to this possibility, some of them have adopted an "If you can't beat 'em, join 'em" approach, adopting holistic practices in varying degrees. The frequent calls for "integration" of holistic and traditional practices may serve the purpose of preserving the hegemony of medicine by co-opting the most attractive components of holism. According to Salmon and Berliner (1980), those M.D.'s who choose to disregard holism will suffer a loss of patients:

> Obviously, physicians hostile to or ignorant of the holistic approach tend to lose out on two counts: not only will holistic-styled practitioners steer people away from them, but the preferences and demands of consumers themselves for more responsive care will lead them to look elsewhere. (p. 245)

Both medicine and nursing claimed to be the natural and necessary leaders of the movement toward the promotion of wellness. Fleming (1980) asserts: "Clearly, we physicians cannot effect a higher state of wellness for the population without the cooperation and effort of all the individuals involved, but just as clearly, we do have responsibility to serve as the leaders" (p. 21). Wooley (1986), on the other hand, claims that nursing is "the right profession to lead the wellness parade" (p. 201).

This jockeying for power and patients has tended to obscure the fact that both nursing and medicine have historically incorporated elements of what is now being referred to as holistic care into their practices. As has been indicated throughout this book, many holistic theses are not only accepted by the conventional health professions, but were originated by them. Vanderpool (1984), in his review of holistic medicine, argues that "the concerns of whole-person care are longstanding and commonly shared (even if not put into practice), and have long been regarded as significant. The new term *holism* seems to trivialize these concerns, rather than to capture or highlight them" (p. 777). As Vanderpool notes, the ideals of holists are sometimes honored in the breach. Nevertheless, their claim that conventional providers abandoned such ideals after Descartes cannot be supported. In particular, efforts have been made to avoid the problems that arise when patients are treated in a de-personalized fashion, as diseases or problems.

Primary nursing, for example, is a system designed to assure that patients have the opportunity to establish a relationship with one professional who assumes responsibility for their nursing care, thus providing for continuity. Primary nursing is described by Marram, Barrett, and Bevis as patient-centered, individualized, and comprehensive: "The primary nurse considers the emotional, psychosocial, spiritual, and physical aspects of patient problems and needs" (1979, p. 51). Although such care is often more a goal than a reality, the need for a less fragmented approach to care has clearly been recognized by the nursing profession.

Similarly, medicine has recognized the need for comprehensive care. One response to the public frustration with care has been the establishment of family practice as a recognized medical specialty (Geyman, 1985). Like primary nursing, family practice is concerned with continuity and comprehensiveness of care, and with a provider-patient relationship that is ongoing and trusting (McWhinney, 1981). According to Geyman, "The shift toward family practice . . . represents a positive step by the medical profession to respond directly to the changing needs of society. This shift can be viewed as one away from primary concern for diseases and organ systems, toward the whole patient as a person, his/her family, and the community" (p. 6).

The growth of primary nursing and of family practice in medicine are but two examples of attempts by conventional providers to provide comprehensive and personal care. Other concerns of holists are addressed by conventional practitioners as well. For example, considerable attention has been given to preventive measures (community health) and to the mind-body relationship (psychosomatic and behavioral medicine). The efforts of conventional practitioners to provide comprehensive, individualized care that is person- rather than disease-oriented have been successful in varying degrees. The failures have been significant enough that many patients continue to experience frustration when dealing with the health-care system. Nevertheless, the efforts of conventional providers in this regard are legitimate and worthy in their own right. For conventional providers to describe their efforts as "holistic" wrongly suggests that they have no relationship to earlier advances in health care and, as Vanderpool suggests, trivializes professional concerns relative to quality of care.

Caring for the Whole Person

Whatever the motivation of the newly holistic provider—political, economic, or the desire to achieve excellence in practice—the common rallying cry is: "We must care for the whole person." The original intent of this slogan was to indicate a concern for more than the disorder, recognition of the patient as a human being, and consideration of nonphysical aspects of disease. After the fashion of most slogans, however, it came to be understood more literally. The term "whole person" is now supposed to denote every characteristic that could possibly be associated with people—not just their minds and bodies, but their roles, problems, and places of work. A person, it seems, no longer stops at the confines of the body, but has expanded to fill an indeterminate space. The expansion of the person has paralleled the expansion of the concept of health. Just as health was seen to become more remote as its definition was enlarged, so too has the possibility of caring for the whole person become more difficult as more meanings have accrued to the concept of personal wholeness. The whole person, in fact, has become a rather unwieldy patient.

The role of the health provider has needed to undergo a corresponding dilation. In conventional medical practice, the practitioner endeavors to assist ill persons to regain good health. But holistic medicine, says Canton (1980), "is a manifestation of the desire for a better quality of life" (p. 171). Dentists, who formerly confined their practice to the mouth and teeth now find that "the dentist is in a position to assist in clarifying lifetime values" (White, 1980, p. 75). When assessing a client for possible problems, holistic practitioners are cautioned against limiting their observations to signs of illness. Flynn advises that, when holistic wellness is assessed, "we are evaluating the human condition" (1980, p. 129).

The amount of data deemed necessary for an adequate assessment by some practitioners can be staggering. Regarding evaluation of the hospitalized patient, Strauss (1978) states:

> Unless these efforts include empathic inquiry into the nature and circumstances of the individual's home life, marital and intra- and extra-familial relationships, work situations, aspirations, and expectations, it will result in a mere sketch of a limited aspect of a human being. (p. 557)

Strauss's conclusion is correct. He does not, however, entertain the possibility that such a limited sketch would provide an adequate, even the most appropriate, data base in many patient-care situations.

Once the mountain of necessary data has been assembled, the practitioner must sort through it to identify problems, which may or may not resemble those typically assigned to the province of health care. No matter. They are problems of the whole person. We *treat* the whole person. Ergo, we must treat all associated problems. This logic has put a tremendous burden on providers, forcing them to assume roles for which they are ill prepared. It is unrealistic to expect an internist to act as a policeman, a nurse to act as a lawyer, or a dentist to act as a social worker.

Granting that economic, social, and environmental in-fluences can adversely affect health, can we also assume that health professionals can or ought to be responsible for ameliorating these conditions or treating the resulting problems? Some would say not. Narayan and Joslin (1980), discussing problems resulting from poverty and slums, question "the 'right' of community health profes-sionals to tamper, on a large scale, with social conditions of such magnitude"(p. 33). Kopelman and Moskop (1981) doubt the feasibility of providing for the patients' total well-being and challenge the expertise of providers in nonhealth areas:

> [Are practitioners] obligated to inquire about how much they enjoy gardening, music, sex, baseball, reading, their families, cooking, hiking, their work, etc.? Are they then obligated to try to do something, for example, to "pre-scribe" Mozart, Chekhov, or belly dancing? Does not this definition of health in terms of well-being lead to an un-realistic expansion of the obligations that providers have in delivering health care to their clients? . . . Perhaps the clients do not care to discuss or be counselled about their working conditions, family, habits, mode of living, and philosophical or religious convictions. What qualifies the health practitioner as a counselor in moral matters about how others ought to live their lives? (pp. 213 and 226)

On one level, this criticism could be countered by not-ing those instances in which knowledge of life-style and personal preferences could be useful in influencing health outcomes. A nurse working with a patient in a cardiac rehabilitation program, for instance, would find it useful to inquire about each of the items listed by Kopelman and Moskop in order to assist the patient in making appropriate choices regarding meal planning, ac-tivity level, and stress management. The authors' actual concern, however, is the drift of health providers away from the health arena into the marginal area of well-being, a consequence, as noted in chapter 3, of enlarging the definition of health.

Time, too, is an issue. Most practitioners feel hard-pressed to attend to the standard health care needs of their patients. How is the general practitioner, who averages thirteen minutes per patient, to find time for whole-person care as defined by the holists (Noren, Frazier, Altman, and DeLozier, 1980)?

Overspecialization and fragmentation of services have been replaced by the opposite problem of care providers who take on too much and make promises they cannot keep. It simply is not possible for one individual to be an expert in recognizing and treating every affliction of mankind, but the holists continue to take on more roles, to assume responsibility for more problems, to try to treat the whole person. One senses a kind of competition among providers to do the most, to care the most, to be, in a sense, "wholier than thou."

Interprofessional sniping breaks out. A nurse:

The medical model encourages doctors and others to view a patient as simply a diseased liver, surrounded by other matter that may or may not be important. This other "ir-relevant" matter may include the patient's psycholog-ic well-being, financial well-being, social situation, spiritual beliefs, and general habits of health care. (Brallier, 1978, pp. 646–647)

A doctor:

Nurses, too, are militantly laying claim to a superior knowledge of and feeling for the patient, some even ar-rogating to themselves the responsibility to protect the

patient from the "cold, insensitive physician." (Engel,
G. L., 1979, p. 264)

Treating the whole patient has become a matter of principle *and* pride. The slogan has calcified and is now interpreted quite literally: the care giver who cares is bound
to search out and treat all problems. It is the most revered
of all holistic statements, and few in or out of the movement dare to challenge it. Pellegrino (1982) observes that
"even the ardent reductionists will pay lip service to the
importance of the 'whole patient' " (p. x).

Still, the question must be asked: Is it possible to care
for the whole person? Perhaps it is possible to be concerned about the whole person; surely there are those
who try to address every problem to some extent. But
certainly no one provider can care for the whole person
as identified by the holists. It is too large a task. "In order
to speak of health," says Paul Tillich, "one must speak
of all dimensions of life which are united in man. And
no one can be an expert in all of them" (1961, p. 92). It
is the rigidness with which holists interpret the whole-
person slogan that impels them to try. Some care givers
refuse that obligation:

> Where in the name of everything holy does it say that a
> physician is to be more than a healer of sick-
> ness? . . . Why in the world are we expected to be all
> things to all people and take care of all of everyone's
> problems? . . . Certainly no one expects a clergyman to
> do appendectomies or a sociologist to treat acute glo-
> merulonephritis. (Friedlieb, 1979, p. 1490)

Friedlieb complains that he should not be *expected* to
take on the burdensome responsibility of meeting all the

patient's needs. G. Francis (1980) offers the more significant insight that in fact it is not *possible* for care givers
to fulfill the demands of such a responsibility. She believes they fool themselves when they are persuaded that
they do so, especially with regard to psychosocial needs.
Any attempt by health-care providers to turn the relationship between themselves and their patients from a
secondary to a primary relationship, she says, will result
in *pseudo-gemeinschaft*—an artificial intimacy. A physical
therapist, for example, might empathize with a patient
grieving over the death of a loved one, but could not
replace the lost relationship and should not claim to be
able to do so:

> A whole person must of necessity become role-fragmen-
> ted, as in a rider to the bus driver and a patient to the
> health worker. . . . Many professional health care work-
> ers could probably do much more for patients . . . but
> they cannot give *total* care. Human needs reach far be-
> yond anyone's or any team's, ability to meet them. (pp.
> 12 and 13)

Noting that in the past decade many nursing schools
have organized their curricula around the concept of holistic care, Clearage (1984) asks: "Is it possible that nursing is expressing its naiveté in attempting to cope with
all aspects of man?" (p. 308).

The holists have set themselves a standard they cannot
meet. It is not possible to care for the whole person. The
notion that practitioners should do so evolved from the
thesis that the whole cannot be understood by examining
its parts. Even if this were true (and I think it can be very
profitable to look at, for example, a spleen), one might
still question the *necessity* of understanding the whole.

The emergency-room nurse who cares for the child who is brought in for suturing of a hand laceration will not only attend to the hand, but will try to allay the child's fears and perhaps do some teaching with the parents regarding household safety. Although the nurse has done more than simply treat the part, in no way has the whole been treated. Were the nurse to discuss every aspect of the child's health and development, the waiting room would soon be filled with angry clients. Instead, professional judgment is used to choose which needs to address. The mind and body, as Heron (1983) points out, do demonstrate functional independence as well as interdependence, a fact "that legitimates some degree of Cartesian dualism in practice" (p. 97).

If we share Morgan's belief that "wholeness does not reside in the individual as an isolated being but in the person who is in relationship with the world" (1968, p. 326), then we must accept that care givers cannot engage in caring for the whole person because that would be an assignment without boundaries.

A Question of Perspective

The question of boundaries and limits is central to the conflict between the holists and conventional providers. The holists claim that medicine (a term that in this section will denote all conventional health-care disciplines) defines its practice too narrowly, an approach that results in de-humanizing treatment of patients. Medicine is accused of focusing on the disease, the part, and the technique—all at the expense, of course, of the "whole person." It is too much concerned, accuse the holists, with the therapy and too little with the patient. The scientific method is felt to impose too small a focus.

Conventional providers, on the other hand, protest that the holists are acting irresponsibly by trying to assign every human problem to the province of health care, thereby increasing the already heavy burden of practitioners. They believe that use of the scientific method allows them to do what they do best—heal the sick—and that holism may be encouraging them to do many things badly.

So we see a clash of perspectives, medicines' being narrowly defined and clearly focused, holism's being global and expansive. Presently, medicine finds itself on the defensive as the holists tout the superiority of their perspective. It is not surprising that more than one perspective should compete for dominance. A perspective, after all, is a way of understanding, ordering, and giving coherence to the phenomena we encounter. Perspective is not bias, though it is a tool that can be used in a biased manner. To be without perspective is not to be without prejudice. Indeed, Schrag (1969) claims that perspectivity is unavoidable. When we are concerned with something so large, complex, and significant as human health, our perspectives allow us to understand and describe it. Without perspective, the task would be overwhelming.

Proponents of a particular perspective may legitimately try to demonstrate—as the holists do—that theirs is a richer or more fruitful or more accurate perspective than a competing one. They must then support that claim.

Some world views *are* arguably better than others. Occasionally it is suggested that sharply differing views are "just a matter of perspective," as if a perspective were insignificant and represented nothing more than a personal proclivity to consider a subject from a particular slant. This interpretation derives from the linear or architectural usage of the term as a view obtainable from a particular position. But the conceptual perspective of a movement, though inclusive of this usage, must be something more. It is a means of seeking and assigning meaning, and it would be foolish to refer to a difference of opinion as "just a matter of meaning."

The holists, of course, are unlikely to underestimate the significance of their perspective. They tend to err in the opposite direction, believing that it is so unique, self-contained, and correct that it disallows the possibility of dialogue with those using other perspectives. This is an example of so-called "point-of-view philosophy," in which persons holding one point of view do not expect to find another intelligible. The consequence and the danger is that perspectives come to be viewed as not subject to criticism from without. One either holds a perspective or does not. If not, then one cannot expect to understand it. Indeed, holists tend to interpret criticism as a failure of comprehension, as if to understand holism is to accept it.

The holists' assertion of superiority rests on the assumption that it is better to conceptualize man as a unitary whole than as an aggregate of integrated parts. This characterization seems useful in some respects. Using the holistic perspective, we seek evidence of unity, integrity, and relationship. Medicine looks at man and sees systems, organs, and cells. It describes physical and chemical occurrences. The charge, of course, is reductionism. But an honest observer must admit that, just as man is seen to be a whole through the holistic perspective, the scientific perspective of medicine reveals his parts. A good perspective does not dictate what we will find. It does, however, limit what we will look at. Reductionism in medicine is helpful insofar as it enables us to examine man's systems and processes; it goes too far if it proposes that man is only those systems and processes.

What the holists have failed to understand is that they also walk a fine line between a useful and a dangerous reductionism. Some kind of wholeness—its nature not yet clearly conceptualized—is evident in man. The holists make a reductionistic error that parallels medicine's when they conclude that man is only the wholeness they observe. To view a person as only some kind of undifferentiated human substance, or worse, as simply a manifestation of the stuff of the universe, is to willfully ignore evidence to the contrary.

Both holism and medicine discuss health from interesting and useful perspectives. It is far from evident that the holistic perspective is the better of the two. But the holists go so far as to proclaim that theirs is not only better, but is the only legitimate one to use relative to questions of health. Further, they believe it to be applicable to other concerns as well because health is seen as related to all of life. Like many other ideologies, holism has been overextended. It is always dangerous to try to explain all occurrences using the perspective of a single system, a practice that tends to promote zeolatry.

We ought to be wary of any "ism" that claims unlimited usefulness. Perhaps the justifiable limits of a system are transgressed when the "ism" begins to produce adherents who identify themselves solely by their allegiance to the world view of that system. A woman may find feminism a useful tool for explaining many political, social, and economic events. If her primary identity is that of feminist, however, she may begin to interpret everything in terms of women's relationship to men. Buchler (1951) has observed that some perspectives of great usefulness have become rigid and authoritarian:

> The character of a perspective is as important as its identity, and it can lend itself to idolatry as well as to exploration. The great faiths of men, the great "schools" of philosophy and art, have been the influential perspectives within which men have been able to attain coherency. They have functioned as quasi-social devices by which query has defined its order and within which it has fed itself. They have also been castles of orthodoxy. Their borders have hardened into impassable fortresses, and the processes of query have dried into vested interests of the spirit. (p. 118)

The vision of the holistic health movement is in grave danger of becoming (may already have become) the kind of orthodoxy that permits of no questioning and allows for no change. It does not guide inquiry so much as announce answers. Little accommodation is made for other perspectives. Instead, holism tries to subsume them within its own. Schrag (1969) warns against attempting to unify multiple perspectives within a single one, contending that this is unacceptable because "it involves an absolutization of a particular standpoint and a particular version of the world, which belies an unspoken claim for absolute knowledge" (p. 280).

The holistic claim to absolute knowledge is not unspoken but is clearly articulated. When a "foreign" concept is found to be valuable, it is simply incorporated; it becomes part of the whole. Other perspectives are not regarded as having their own integrity and usefulness, but as either misconceived or actually a part of holism that has been dissected away.

Schrag goes on to claim that "franchises must be granted to the multiple ways of speaking about the world" (p. 280). This does not suggest that one way is as good as another or that tolerance must be exercised in hearing out wrong-headed ideas. It does indicate that a single world view can never constitute a perfect image of reality. We ought to entertain multiple ways of speaking about the world because they may have something to teach us. A perspective tested against others may be revealed as faulty or inadequate, or its strengths may stand out more clearly. It may actually be enriched or enlarged by the encounter. But a perspective like holism's, which has pretensions to absolute knowledge, does not change or grow, but remains fixed within its boundaries.

Perspectives have been described by Schrag as having both subjective and objective aspects; that is, a perspective is both solicited by what is observed as well as projected by the observer. If the objective reality of a particular terrain is fixed, the subjective is not, or need not be. It is the subjective aspect that allows and even demands the tolerance of multiple perspectives. Thus, the holists may try to argue that theirs is a good perspective, but not that it is the *only* legitimate perspective.

The use of the term "subjective" does not here imply point-of-view subjectivism, for, as Buchler notes, perspectives can be shared, adopted, and divided. Rather than assuming that they are in possession of the only accurate understanding of health, holists might consider in what ways their perspective is particularly illuminating and to what tasks it is best suited. What other perspectives might enrich their own? Conventional medicine, too, ought to ask these questions of itself. Holism and conventional medicine need not consider themselves as engaged in a dispute only one can win. Nor do these groups have the only perspectives useful for considering questions of health. Some religious traditions, for example, offer insights into these questions.

If perspectives can, in fact, be shared, then holism and conventional medicine each could benefit by exploring the other's world and evaluating the possibilities it offers its own. And, if a perspective may be divided without being destroyed, providers could incorporate selected aspects of one into their own practice, or use it only occasionally.

Unfortunately, it is not a simple matter for a person educated and practicing in a particular tradition to adopt or borrow part or all of another perspective, however appealing. It is not that professions merely become stubborn or narrow-minded or set in their ways. Certain habits of mind become part of the very structure of a profession and, for its practitioners, have tremendous influence on the way they view the world. Bensman and Lilienfeld (1973) have argued that not only the professions but also every occupation or craft inevitably contributes to the formation of characteristic attitudes and ways of thinking in its practitioners.

In time, these habits of mind may become so thoroughly assimilated that they are no longer identified as part of a particular perspective: "It is unfortunate that individuals who start their work with self-consciously created points of reference lose, in the process of doing the work, their awareness that they are viewing only a limited aspect of the world" (p. 349). It is, in other words, difficult to maintain an awareness of perspective as such. When the habitual perspective of an occupation is no longer consciously identified, it is no longer available for evaluation. The risk of perspective becoming rigid orthodoxy is decreased when practitioners can observe their habits of mind with some detachment and ask if they are adequate to the tasks of the profession.

But perspective also helps a profession to determine which tasks it ought to undertake. The complaint of the holists is that conventional providers have defined their tasks too narrowly; this is the essence of the whole-person argument. Some providers dismiss the idea that they could or ought to be doing more than what the practice of their profession traditionally entails, but others are stung by the accusations of holists and patients. They acknowledge the limitations of their perspective and wonder if perhaps the holists are not onto something. They recognize that the traditional professions are rigid in some ways, locked into certain habits of mind that may prevent them from attending effectively to the human needs of their patients. The constraints of a disease-oriented system are felt to be unacceptably limiting. Some truth is noted in the charges of insensitivity, arrogance, and narrow-mindedness.

Various practitioners have begun to consider the questions Kestenbaum (1982) poses: "What maximally, not minimally, is the work of the nurse, physician, occupational and physical therapist? What habits of mind previously considered 'merely' desirable have become morally compelling for the responsible health professional who wishes to grasp the intelligibility of illness on a human, as well as technical, level?" (pp. 12–13). As care givers search for answers to these questions, they may begin to feel that their profession has used a minimal interpretation of its work that they can no longer defend. The holistic alternative may seem promising, but its interpretation of the maximal work of the health professional is flawed.

Still, the holistic perspective may offer some insight to

the conventional professions as they struggle to reassess their practices. They need not jettison their own perspectives in order to investigate another. Unfortunately, the holists, with typical excess, have insisted that their view of the world is a package that must be adopted in its entirety or not at all. (This claim is common among movements purporting to be in possession of a superior perspective.)

But they have probably done themselves a disservice. Professionals are likely to resist. Occupational habits of mind are not readily modified or abandoned, nor should they be. Perspectives change only gradually and by increments. Practitioners may be intrigued by some, but not all, holistic ideas. As Buchler states, "It is possible to reject a philosophic assertion while accepting a total perspective, and possible to reject a perspective while isolating and accepting an assertion. But more than that: it is possible to accept part of a perspective"(p. 123). Both holists and conventional practitioners could benefit if the holists were willing to share, not impose, their perspective.

Conventional practitioners, for their part, need not become holists in order to make use of the holistic perspective. Perhaps the practitioner does not care for the whole person, but for the person who is whole. The holistic perspective may help identify ways in which part of a person can be treated without injuring human integrity, or wholeness. The holists' conception of health and their understanding of the responsibilities of practitioners are broad. They can serve as a reminder to those employing the narrower focus of conventional medicine that multiple perspectives are available. A broad perspective, however, is not necessarily a deep or profound perspective and may be less compelling than one that is smaller but richer. The holists have not increased the power of their perspective by enlarging the scope of what it considers. The effect is simply additive—confusing and not clarifying.

Summary

Health professionals have not been able to ignore the holistic health movement. The public has found conventional care, though technically competent, to be inadequate. The response on the part of some practitioners has been to champion the holistic alternative. But the grandiose solutions of the holists have posed their own problems. If technical competence is not enough, and caring for the whole person is too much, then what constitutes good care? Holism is an excessive response, but it is a response to real problems. The problems themselves cannot be dismissed because the solution is found wanting. The answer to this question does not involve finding the correct point on a continuum of services. Rather, it requires the health professions to consider carefully the nature of their obligations to their patients and to identify perspectives that will assist them in this effort.

The assertion of the holists that they possess the only such perspective is not justified. Could it be that the movement would achieve more success by reducing its ambitions? Rather than claiming the ultimate perspective for dealing with issues of health, it could more modestly suggest that it is one of several useful perspectives. Holists could, like William James, "stand out for the legitimacy of the notion of *some*. . . . '' In some settings, for some persons, facing some problems, the holistic approach may be the most fruitful. In some instances, it may be inappropriate. And, in many instances, it may be best to include holism as one among several perspectives.

Conclusion

Even those who find some merit in the arguments that have been presented against holism may be tempted to shrug and ask "so what?" They may think that holism, though it is presently attracting considerable attention, is merely a trend that is already beginning to pass from the scene. Perhaps holism will go the way of one of its forebears, the counterculture, fading into the past and only occasionally recalled, albeit with some affection, as an aberrant phenomenon. This may well occur. The term "holistic" may, in a few years, sound as quaint as "commune" does today.

This possibility does not justify disregarding the movement, however. The movement may die, but it will not vanish without a trace. Ideas, attitudes, beliefs—all of which influence practice—will remain. Gillette (1980), in discussing holism, notes that "social movements often contain a mixture of truths which endure, unsound components which fall in time of their own weight, and a tendency for a few of their adherents to carry rational ideas to irrational extremes" (p. 1093). I have argued that many holistic tenets are unsound. Yet, they show no signs of "falling by their own weight." Rather, they have gained credibility. Gillette is too sanguine in assuming that the wheat and the chaff of holism will separate naturally over time. The wave of popularity the movement is experiencing is giving buoyancy to good and bad ideas alike.

What accounts for this popularity? Why have so many persons, so many groups, become enchanted with holism? How is it that its quasi-scientific model has become such a force? The previous chapter pointed out that the holistic health movement has commanded attention by focusing on problems that have been ignored or handled badly within the conventional system of health care. The holists are keenly aware of the frustration with the limitations of that system.

Another of the movement's major attractions is the sense of control it provides. Adherents are encouraged to believe that there are therapies, behaviors, and attitudes that must inevitably contribute to a state of well-being. Great satisfaction is taken in doing the right thing. When the correct behavior is followed by good health, patients may take pride in their belief that the relationship is causal. Holists rely heavily on the "if only" technique. If only we meditated twice a day, we would not be at-risk for migraine headaches. The "if only" technique provides a sense of control; it also suggests that satisfaction can be taken in doing the right thing. The pleasures of self-righteousness play no small part in holistic health.

Finally, the movement is attractive because its scheme is purported to be both comprehensive and simple. It deals not only with health, but also with the entire human condition. Simple answers are available, the holists suggest, to problems that have been regarded as overwhelmingly complex. It has answers to health problems, yes, but it also offers insights into philosophical problems, social dilemmas, environmental concerns, and spiritual issues. Advocates then, do not feel it can be adequately described as merely a health-care system; therefore, such terms as philosophy, orientation, and perspective are used. Holism may be regarded as a kind of world view. It is a comprehensive system claiming to be capable of explaining all phenomena. Its appeal lies in its simplicity. There is no need to deal with ambiguity or with conflicting values, no need to struggle with the problems of human suffering that have long bedeviled us. Every concern of man lends itself to holistic analysis and resolution.

Certainly it is not unusual for a movement that has identified deficiencies in the prevailing system to achieve rapid ascendancy, especially when it assumes the characteristics of a world view. Marxism offers an example of such a world view. The troubles of the working class were clearly identified, and a system was constructed to address them. Members of the movement began to apply Marxist solutions to any number of woes: political, social, economic. Just as Marxists use the concept of class, holists use the concept of human wholeness as the lens through which the world is viewed. Comprehensive systems or world views that achieve wide popularity and acquire many adherents tend to produce ideas that find their way out of the confines of the movement and into the cultural consciousness. Persons who do not regard themselves as Marxists or Freudians may be heard discussing class struggle or the ego.

So it is with holism. Those who are influenced by its thinking may be divided into three groups. In the first are the true believers. For these individuals, an appreciation of the virtues of holism comes with the immediacy and impact of revelation. They may have undergone a personal healing experience, or may simply have been struck by what they perceive to be the obvious truth and clarity of holistic thought. The second group includes those who have been recruited into the movement, perhaps after a period of initial skepticism. The recruit may have been propagandized by one or more true believers and has come to believe that the holistic approach offers many advantages. This group includes many conventional health-care providers. Lastly, there are many outside the movement who do not consider themselves holists, but who are, nevertheless, profoundly influenced by the ideas of the movement. They may be committed, for example, to the belief that they are responsible for their own health, though they do not recognize the holistic roots of this notion.

Thus, the influence of holism has been more extensive than is generally realized. Were it not for the impact it has had on nonholists, the movement might be dismissed as silly but harmless. But, as has happened with other sweeping systems, holistic ideas have insinuated themselves into our everyday dialogue. At this level, they may become diluted or distorted. They may be interpreted more concretely. According to Bensman and Lilienfeld (1973), "The attitudes of everyday life are a simplified, vulgarized, de-intellectualized reflection of highly articulated systems of thought originally developed by intellectuals, and disseminated through the communication machinery of a society" (p. 344). One could never support the claim that the present holistic movement was created by intellectuals or that it represents a highly articulated system of thought.

It is necessary to go one step further back in its history and recall that the movement drew its inspiration from thinkers in religion, philosophy, psychology, and other areas. If the Bensman-Lilienfeld analysis is correct, then we can assume that the ideas propounded early in the life of the modern holistic health movement themselves represented a vulgarization of others' thoughts on human wholeness. In a reverse of the usual route of transmission, these ideas then found their way back into the discourse of professionals and intellectuals. Persons in these groups adopted many of the notions of the holists and tried to put a little intellectual and/or scientific shine on them. Physicians were heard talking more about the importance of prevention, and prominent lay people such as Norman Cousins stressed the value of natural therapies. "Holism" entered the professional lexicon. The approval of health professionals, particularly, gave authority and credibility to holistic ideas. Individuals who might have dismissed the recommendations of a self-styled holistic healer were more receptive to the same prescriptions when they were refashioned as a physician's order.

The ideology of the movement, then, is at three removes from the original source of its inspiration; and, each time holistic ideas are passed along to another group, they become, as Bensman and Lilienfeld observe, further simplified, vulgarized, and de-intellectualized, until they are compressed into the familiar slogans.

It is in this form that holistic thought is adopted by nonholists and finds its way into the fabric of conventional wisdom. Although proponents of holism are easily identified and their arguments stated at least clearly enough to be challenged, the unconscious absorption of holistic notions—a kind of cultural osmosis—is more pervasive, more difficult to identify, and less likely to be challenged. Holistic ideas are especially difficult to evaluate because they come to us capsulized in statements that, on some level, have value. If the deeper meanings and possibilities are ignored, they are difficult to refute.

Half-truths are the powerful medium for the transmission of holistic ideology. The most poisonous ideas are sometimes those that appear self-evidently worthy.

This may explain the virtual absence of rigorous critical evaluation the movement has enjoyed to date. It is remarkable how little serious discussion has been occasioned by its tenets and the significant claims made on their behalf. The criticism that has been offered could be characterized as generally superficial and frequently involves merely a rejection, not an evaluation, of the tenets. This book began with Lovejoy's observation that whole generations may be dominated by types of thinking that may "amount to a large and important and perhaps highly debatable proposition." Holism, although highly debatable, is little debated.

If the holistic health movement has made a significant contribution, it lies in its articulation of the problems and not in its proposed solutions. Holists, however, repeatedly make the mistake of confusing the two. Does fragmentation of services leave patients feeling helpless and frustrated? Simply recognize this and "treat the whole person." But this is a restatement, not a resolution, of the problem. It does allow us to believe in the availability of simple remedies. If certain practices in health care present problems, all that is necessary is to stop doing them. The leap from assessment to intervention has been made too quickly; the answers are too glib. The holists would do well to return to the original health-care problems that have interested them and carefully consider how they might be approached.

If they are to defend their movement successfully against the criticism that must surely be offered in the future, they will need to provide a more fully realized theory to replace the slogans now in use. Some of their ideas have value but are superficial and require refinement. Others are faulty and ought to be discarded. If the holists want to be given serious consideration, they will have to allow their perspective to be investigated and evaluated, and must be willing to engage in serious debate about its merits, acknowledging that it will not be accepted all-of-a-piece as it has been presented. Finally, they will need to moderate their claims, which are excessive in the extreme. These are tough demands to make of a movement that has been notable for its evangelical enthusiasm since its inception. If the holists take no responsibility for meeting them, they may see their formal movement die, leaving behind a legacy of unsound ideas.

Bibliography

Ader, R. Psychosomatic and psychoimmunologic research. *Psychosomatic Medicine*, 1980, 42 (3), 307–321.

Agras, W. S. Behavioral medicine in the 1980's: Nonrandom connections. *Journal of Consulting and Clinical Psychology*, 1982, *50* (6), 797–803.

Albright, P. Orthodox Western medicine in the holistic era. In P. Albright and B. P. Albright (Eds.), *Body, mind, and spirit*. Brattleboro, Vermont: The Stephen Greene Press, 1980a.

————. Using inner and outer resources. In P. Albright and B. P. Albright (Eds.), *Body, mind, and spirit*. Brattleboro, Vermont: The Stephen Greene Press, 1980b.

Albright, P., and Albright, B. P. Introduction. In P. Albright and B. P. Albright (Eds.), *Body, mind, and spirit*. Brattleboro, Vermont: The Stephen Greene Press, 1980.

Alexander, A. B. Asthma. In S. N. Haynes and L. G. Gannon, (Eds.), *Psychosomatic disorders*. New York: Praeger Publishers, 1981.

Alp, M. H., Court, J. H., and Grant, A. K. Personality pattern and emotional stress in the genesis of gastric ulcer. *Gut*, 1970, *11* (9), 773–777.

Angell, M. Disease as a reflection of the psyche. *The New England Journal of Medicine*, 1985, *312*, (24), 1570–1572.

Ansbacher, H. L. On the origin of holism. *Journal of Individual Psychology*, 1961, *17* (2), 142–148.

Apple, D. How laymen define illness. *Journal of Health and Human Behavior*, 1960, 1 (3), 219–225.

Aral, S. O., Cates, W., and Jenkins, W. C. Genital herpes: Does knowledge lead to action? *American Journal of Public Health*, 1985, 75 (1), 69–71.

Ardell, D. High-level wellness and the HSA's: A health-planning success story. *American Journal of Health Planning*, 1978, 3 (3), 1–18.

Aristotle. [*De Anima*] (D. Ross, Ed. and Trans.). London: Oxford at the Clarendon Press, 1961.

———. *Aristotle's Metaphysics* (H. G. Apostle, Trans.). Grinnell, Iowa: The Peripatetic Press, 1979.

Asterita, M. F. *The physiology of stress*. New York: Human Sciences Press, Inc., 1985.

Baric, L. Recognition of the "at-risk" role: A means to influence health behaviour. *International Journal of Health Education*, 1969, 12 (1), 24–34.

Beaber, R. J. Stress—And other scapegoats. *Newsweek*, April 4, 1983, p. 13.

Becker, E. *The structure of evil*. New York: George Braziller, 1968.

Becker, M. H. Understanding patient compliance: The contributions of attitudes and other psychosocial factors. In S. J. Cohen (Ed.), *New directions in patient compliance*. Lexington, Massachusetts: D. C. Heath and Company, 1979.

Beland, I. L. (Ed.). *Clinical nursing: Pathophysiological and psychosocial approaches* (2nd ed.). New York: The Macmillan Company, 1970.

Belloc, N. B. Relationship of health practices and mortality. *Preventive Medicine*, 1973, 2 (1), 67–81.

Belloc, N. B., and Breslow, L. Relationship of physical health status and health practices. *Preventive Medicine*, 1972, 1 (3), 409–421.

Bensman, J., and Lilienfeld, R. *Craft and consciousness*. New York: John Wiley & Sons, 1973.

Benson, H. *The relaxation response*. New York: William Morrow, 1975.

————. *The mind/body effect*. New York: Berkley Books/Simon and Schuster, 1979.

Berg, A. O. Adult health maintenance in family practice: A ten-year reassessment. *The Journal of Family Practice*, 1986, *22* (4), 319–320.

Bergman, A. B. and Werner, R. J. Failure of children to receive penicillin by mouth. *The New England Journal of Medicine*, 1963, *268* (24), 1334–1338.

Bergsma, J., and Thomasma, D. C. *Health care: Its psychosocial dimensions*. Pittsburgh: Dusquesne University Press, 1982.

Berkeley Holistic Health Center. *The holistic health handbook*. Berkeley, California: And/Or Press, 1978.

Berlin, I. *Against the current: Essays in the history of ideas* (H. Hardy, Ed.). New York: The Viking Press, 1980.

Berliner, H. S., and Salmon, J. W. The holistic alternative to scientific medicine: History and analysis. *International Journal of Health Services*, 1980, *10* (1), 133–147.

Besson, G. The health-illness spectrum. *American Journal of Public Health*, 1967, *57* (11), 1901–1905.

Betz, T. G. Conflicts in the study of Chagas' disease between a southwestern Indian population and the staff of a southwestern university college of medicine. In E. E. Bauwens (Ed.), *The anthropology of health*. St. Louis: The C. V. Mosby Company, 1978.

Bieliauskas, L. A. *Stress and its relationship to health and illness*. Boulder, Colorado: Westview Press, 1982.

Blaszczynski, A. P. Personality factors in classical migraine and tension headache. *Headache*, 1984, *24* (5), 238–244.

Block, M. B. Holistic medicine: Is it all good? (Editorial). *Arizona Medicine*, 1981, *38* (5), 380.

Blotcky, A. D., and Tittler, B. I. Psychosocial predictors of physical illness: Toward a holistic model of health. *Preventive Medicine*, 1982, *11* (5), 602–611.

Boyd, P. *The silent wound*. Reading, Massachusetts: Addison-Wesley Publishing Company, 1984.

Brallier, L. W. The nurse as holistic health practitioner. *The Nursing Clinics of North America*, 1978, *13* (4), 643–655.

Brandt, P. A. Two different worlds . . . The Navajo child's

interactions within the health care system. In M. Leininger (Ed.), *Transcultural nursing*. New York: John Wiley & Sons, 1978.

Breslow, L. A quantitative approach to the World Health Organization definition of health: Physical, mental and social well-being. *International Journal of Epidemiology*, 1972 1 (4), 347–355.

————. A policy assessment of preventive health practice. *Preventive Medicine*, 1977, 6 (2), 242–251.

Bridgman, R. F. Traditional Chinese medicine. In J. Z. Bowers and E. F. Purcell (Eds.), *Medicine and society in China*. Philadelphia: Josiah Macy, Jr., Foundation, 1974.

Brown, V. A. From sickness to health: An altered focus for health-care research. *Social Science & Medicine*, 1981, 15A, 195–201.

Buchler, J. *Toward a general theory of human judgement*. New York: Columbia University Press, 1951.

Buck, C., and Hobbs, G. E. The problem of specificity in psychosomatic illness. In M. L. Hirt (Ed.), *Psychological and allergic aspects of asthma*. Springfield, Illinois: Charles C. Thomas Publisher, 1965.

Burrow, J. G. *Organized medicine in the progressive era*. Baltimore: The Johns Hopkins University Press, 1977.

Burstein, A. G. What the (w)hole is hellism? (Editorial). *The Pharos*, 1979, 42 (4), 31.

Caldwell, J. Ubiquitous ulcers. *The Boston Globe*, August 1, 1983, p. 34.

Califano, J. *America's health care revolution*. New York: Random House, 1986.

Callahan, D. Health and society: Some ethical imperatives. In J. H. Knowles (Ed.), *Doing better and feeling worse*. New York: W. W. Norton & Company, Inc., 1977.

————. The WHO definition of 'health.' *The Hastings Center Studies*, 1973, 1 (3), 77–87.

Callan, J. P. Holistic health or holistic hoax? (Editorial). *Journal of the American Medical Association*, 1979, 241 (11), 1156.

Canton, R. Holistic medicine: Reactivation of an old aspiration. *The Western Journal of Medicine*, 1980, 133 (2), 171–172.

Capra, F. *The Turning Point*. New York: Simon and Schuster, 1982.

Carey, R. G., and Posovac, E. J. Holistic care in a cancer care center. *Nursing Research*, 1979, *28* (4), 213–216.

Carlson, R. J. Holism and reductionism as perspectives in medicine and health care. *The Western Journal of Medicine*, 1979, *131* (6), 466–470.

————. The future of health care in the United States. In A. C. Hastings, J. Fadiman, and J. S. Gordon (Eds.), *Health for the whole person*. New York: Bantam Books, 1981.

Case, R. B., Heller, S. S., Case, N. B., Moss, A. J., and the Multicenter Post-Infarction Research Group. Type A behavior and survival after acute myocardial infarction. *The New England Journal of Medicine*, 1985, *312* (12), 737–741.

Cassel, E. J. The nature of suffering and the goals of medicine. *The New England Journal of Medicine*, 1982, *306* (11), 639–645.

Cassileth, B. R., Lusk, E. J., Miller, D. S., Brown, L. L., and Miller, C. Psychosocial correlates of survival in advanced malignant disease? *The New England Journal of Medicine*, 1985, *312* (24), 1551–1555.

Chesney, A. P., and Gentry, W. D. Psychosocial factors mediating health risk: A balanced perspective. *Preventive Medicine*, 1982, *11* (5), 612–617.

Chinn, P. L. From the editor. *Advances in Nursing Science*, 1980, 2 (4), xiii.

Christie, M. J. Foundations of psychosomatics. In M. J. Christie and P. G. Mellett (Eds.), *Foundations of psychosomatics*. New York: John Wiley & Sons, 1981.

Clearage, D. K. An integrated curriculum: Idealism or pragmatism? *Journal of Nursing Education*, 1984, *23* (7), 308–310.

Cmich, D. E. Theoretical perspectives of holistic health. *Journal of School Health*, 1984, *54* (1), 30–32.

Cobb, S. Contained hostility in rheumatoid arthritis. *Arthritis and Rheumatism*, 1959, 2 (5), 419–425.

Commins, W. D. Some early holistic psychologists. *The Journal of Philosophy*, 1932, *29* (8), 208–217.

Connolly, J. Life events before myocardial infarction. *Journal of Human Stress*, 1976, 2 (4), 3–17.

Cousins, N. *Anatomy of an illness*. New York: Bantam Books, 1981.

Crawford, R. Healthism and the medicalization of everyday life. *International Journal of Health Services*, 1980, *10* (3), 365–388.

Cunningham, A. J. Should we investigate psychotherapy for physical disease, especially cancer? In S. M. Levy (Ed.), *Biological mediators of behavior and disease: Neoplasia*. New York: Elsevier Science Publishing Co., Inc., 1982.

Davies, N. E. Holistic health care, high-level wellness and the abolition of dis-ease. Editorial. *Southern Medical Journal*, 1979, *72* (11), 1357–1358.

De Luca, J. C. The ulcerative colitis personality. *Nursing Clinics of North America*, 1970, *5* (1), 23–34.

Dewey, J. The reflex arc concept in psychology. *The Psychological Review*, 1896, *3*, 357–370.

———. *Philosophy and civilization*. Gloucester, Massachusetts: Peter Smith, 1968.

———. The unity of the human being. In J. Ratner (Ed.), *Intelligence in the modern world*. New York: Random House, Inc., 1939.

Diamant, A. Matter of mind. *The Boston Phoenix*, May 11, 1982, pp. 1, 8, 10, 12.

Dine, C. *Boston Sunday Globe*, May 30, 1982, pp. 49, 51.

Dock, L. L., and Stewart, I. M. *A short history of nursing* (4th ed.). New York: G. P. Putnam's Sons, 1938.

Dohrenwend, B. S., and Dohrenwend, B. P. Life stress and illness: Formulation of the issues. In their *Stressful life events and their contexts*. New Brunswick, New Jersey: Rutgers University Press, 1984.

Dossey, L. Consciousness and health: What's it all about? *Topics in Clinical Nursing*, 1982, *3* (4), 1–6.

Dubos, R. *Mirage of health*. New York: Harper & Brothers, Publishers, 1959.

———. Hippocrates in modern dress. In D. S. Sobel (Ed.), *Ways of health*. New York: Harcourt, Brace, Jovanovich, 1979a.

————. Preface. In D. S. Sobel (Ed.), *Ways of health*. New York: Harcourt, Brace, Jovanovich, 1979b.

————. Health and creative adaptation. In P. A. R. Flynn (Ed.), *The healing continuum*. Bowie, Maryland: Robert J. Brady Co., 1980.

Duhl, L. J. Holistic health and medicine: A challenge. *The Western Journal of Medicine*, 1979, *131* (6), 473–474.

Dunbar, F. *Mind and body: Psychosomatic medicine*. New York: Random House, 1947–1948.

Dunn, H. L. *High-level wellness*. Virginia: R. W. Beatty, Ltd., 1961.

————. High-level wellness for man and society. *American Journal of Public Health*, 1959, *49* (6), 786–792.

————. Points of attack for raising the levels of wellness. *Journal of the National Medical Association*, 1957, *49* (6), 225–235, 211.

Edlund, M. (Letter). *The New England Journal of Medicine*, 1983, *309* (13), 800.

Eisenberg, L. Disease and illness: Distinctions between professional and popular ideas of sickness. *Culture, Medicine, and Psychiatry*, 1977, *1* (1), 9–23.

————. What makes persons "patients" and patients "well?" *The American Journal of Medicine*, 1980, *69*, 277–286.

Engel, E. Of male bondage. *Newsweek*, June 21, 1982, p. 13.

Engel, G. L. A unified concept of health and disease. *Perspectives in Biology and Medicine*, 1960 *3* (4), 459–485.

————. The biomedical model: A Procrustean bed? *Man and Medicine*, 1979, *4* (4), 257–275.

Engelhardt, H. T. The concepts of health and disease. In A. L. Caplan, H. T. Engelhardt, and J. J. McCartney (Eds.), *Concepts of health and disease*. Reading, Massachusetts: Addison Wesley Publishing Company, 1981.

Engleman, S. R., and Forbes, J. F. Economic aspects of health education. *Social Science & Medicine*, 1986, *22* (4), 443–458.

Feild, L., and Winslow, E. H. Moving to a nursing model. *American Journal of Nursing*, 1985, *85* (10), 1100–1101.

Ferguson, M. *The aquarian conspiracy*. Los Angeles: J. P. Tarcher, Inc., 1980.

Ferguson, T. Medical self-care: Self-responsibility for health. In P. A. R. Flynn (Ed.), *The healing continuum*. Bowie, Maryland: Robert J. Brady Co., 1980.

Fink, D. Holistic health: The evolution of Western medicine. In P. A. R. Flynn (Ed.), *The healing continuum*. Bowie, Maryland: Robert J. Brady Co., 1980.

Fiore, N. Fighting cancer: One patient's perspective. *The New England Journal of Medicine*, 1979, *300* (6), 284–289.

Fleming, T. C. Wellness. *Postgraduate Medicine*, 1980, *67* (2), 19–21.

Flynn, P. A. R. *Holistic health*. Bowie, Maryland: Robert J. Brady Co., 1980.

Foster, G. M., and Anderson, B. G. *Medical anthropology*. New York: John Wiley & Sons, 1978.

Fox, B. H. Premorbid psychological factors as related to cancer incidence. *Journal of Behavioral Medicine*, 1978, *1* (1), 45–133.

Fox, R. C. The medicalization and demedicalization of American society. In J. H. Knowles (Ed.), *Doing better and feeling worse*. New York: W. W. Norton & Company, Inc., 1977.

Frame, P. S. A critical review of adult health maintenance. Part 1: Prevention of atherosclerotic diseases. *The Journal of Family Practice*, 1986, *22* (4), 341–346.

———. A critical review of adult health maintenance. Part 2: Prevention of infectious diseases. *The Journal of Family Practice*, 1986, *22* (5), 417–422.

———. A critical review of adult health maintenance. Part 3: Prevention of cancer. *The Journal of Family Practice*, 1986, *22* (6), 511–520.

———. A critical review of adult health maintenance. Part 4: Prevention of metabolic, behavioral, and miscellaneous conditions. *The Journal of Family Practice*, 1986, *23* (1), 29–39.

Francis, D. P., and Chin, J. The prevention of acquired immunodeficiency syndrome in the United States. *Journal of the American Medical Association*, 1987, *257* (10), 1357–1366.

Francis, G. Gesellschaft and the hospital: Is total care a misnomer? *Advances in Nursing Science*, 1980, *2* (4), 9–13.

Frank, J. D. Holistic medicine: A view from the fence. *The Johns Hopkins Medical Journal*, 1981, *149* (6), 222–227.

Frankl, V. E. *Man's search for meaning*. New York: Pocket Books, 1963.

Freedman, S. A. Megacorporate health care. *The New England Journal of Medicine*, 1985, *312* (9), 579–582.

Friedlieb, O. P. (Letter). *Journal of the American Medical Association*, 1979, *242* (14), 1490.

Friedman, M., and Rosenman, R. H. Association of specific overt behavior pattern with blood and cardiovascular findings. *Journal of the American Medical Association*, 1959, *169* (12), 1286–1296.

Friedman, M., and Ulmer, D. *Treating type-A behavior and your heart*. New York: Alfred A. Knopf, 1984.

Galdston, I. Psychosomatic medicine. In M. L. Hirt (Ed.), *Psychological and allergic aspects of asthma*. Springfield, Illinois: Charles C. Thomas Publisher, 1965.

Galen. *On the natural faculties* (A. J. Brock, Ed. and trans.). Cambridge, Massachusetts: Harvard University Press, 1952.

Gentry, W. D., Chesney, A. P., Gary, H. E., Hall, R. P., and Harburg, E. Habitual anger-coping styles: I. Effect on mean blood pressure and risk for essential hypertension. *Psychosomatic Medicine*, 1982, *44* (2), 195–202.

Geyman, J. P. *Family Practice: Foundation of changing health care* (2nd ed.). Norwalk, Connecticut: Appleton-Century-Crofts, 1985.

Gillette, R. D. Holistic medicine, wellness, and family medicine. *The Journal of Family Practice*, 1980, *10* (6), 1093.

Ginzberg, E. *American medicine*. Totowa, New Jersey: Rowman & Allanheld, 1985.

Glickman, L. Fighting cancer: The patient's perspective (Letter). *The New England Journal of Medicine*, 1979, *300* (21), 1219.

Goldman, L., and Cook, E. F. The decline in ischemic heart disease mortality rates. *Annals of Internal Medicine*, 1984, *101* (6), 825–836.

Goldstein, K. *The organism*. New York: American Book Company, 1939.

Gordon, J. S. The paradigm of holistic medicine. In A. C. Hastings, J. Fadiman, and J. S. Gordon (Eds.), *Health for the whole person*. New York: Bantam Books, 1981.

Gorsuch, R. L., and Key, M. K. Abnormalities of pregnancy as a function of anxiety and life stress. *Psychosomatic Medicine*, 1974, *36* (4), 352–362.

Gottschalk, L. A. Psychosomatic medicine today: An overview. *Psychosomatics*, 1978, *19* (2), 89–93.

Greene, C. S. Holistic dentistry: Where does the holistic end and the quackery begin? *Journal of the American Dental Association*, 1981, *102* (1), 25–27.

Griffith, R. M. Anthropodology: Man a-foot. In S. F. Spicker (Ed.), *The philosophy of the body: Rejections of Cartesian dualism*. Chicago: Quadrangle Books, 1970.

Groen, J. J. The challenge of the future: The prevention of psychosomatic disorders. *Psychotherapy and Psychosomatics*, 1974, *23*, 283–303.

Guttmacher, S. Whole in body, mind, and spirit: Holistic health and the limits of medicine. *The Hastings Center Report*, 1979, *9* (2), 16–21.

Haldane, E., and Ross, G. R. T. *The philosophical works of Descartes* (2 vols.). New York: Cambridge at The University Press, 1968.

Hall, C. S., and Lindzey, G. *Theories of personality* (2nd ed.). New York: John Wiley & Sons, Inc., 1970.

Harmer, B., and Henderson, V. *Textbook of the principles and practice of nursing* (5th ed.). New York: The Macmillan Company, 1955.

Hastings, A. C., Fadiman, J., and Gordon, J. S. (Eds.). *Health for the whole person*. New York: Bantam Books, Inc., 1981.

Haynes, B. R. Improving patient compliance: An empirical view. In R. B. Stuart (Ed.), *Adherence, compliance, and generalization in behavioral medicine*. New York:. Brunner/Mazel, Publishers, 1982.

Hegel, G. W. F. [*Science of logic*] (J. H. Muirhead, Ed.; W. H. Johnston and L. G. Struthers, Trans.). New York: The Macmillan Company, 1929.

Henderson, G., and Primeaux, M. *Transcultural health care*. Menlo Park, California: Addison-Wesley Publishing Company, 1981.

Heron J. Holistic medicine: A cooperative inquiry. *Journal of the Royal Society of Medicine*, 1983, *76* (2), 97–98.

Higgins, C. W. Evaluating wellness programs. *Health Values*, 1986, *10* (6), 44–51.

Hippocrates. *The genuine works of Hippocrates* (F. Adams, Trans.). London: Báillere, Tindall & Cox, 1939.

Holden, C. Cousins' account of self-care rapped. *Science*, 1981, *214* (2), 892.

Holmes, T. H., and Rahe, R. H. The social readjustment rating scale. *Journal of Psychosomatic Research*, 1967, *11* (2), 213–218.

Horn, D. A model for the study of personal choice health behavior. *International Journal of Health Education*, 1976, *19* (2), 89–98.

Horrobin, D. F. *Medical hubris: A reply to Ivan Illich*. Montreal: Eden Press, 1977.

Hubbard, P., Muhlenkamp, A. F., and Brown, N. The relationship between social support and self-care practices. *Nursing Research*, 1984, *33* (5), 266–270.

Illich, I. *Medical nemesis*. New York: Bantam Books, 1977a.

———. *Toward a history of needs*. New York: Pantheon Books, 1977b.

Imperato, P. J., and Mitchell, G. *Acceptable risks*. New York: Viking Penguin, Inc., 1985.

Jacobs, A. D. Holistic health care. *International Journal of Orthodontics*, 1981, *19* (4), 15–16.

James, W. *The principles of psychology* (2 vols.). New York: Dover Publications, Inc., 1950.

———. In R. B. Perry (Ed.), *William James: "Pragmatism" and four essays from "The meaning of truth."* New York: The New American Library, 1974.

———. In J. J. McDermott (Ed.), *The writings of William James*. Chicago: The University of Chicago Press, 1977.

JCO interviews Dr. C. Norman Shealy on holistic health, Part 1. *Journal of Clinical Orthodontics*, 1981, 15 (8), 536–542, 547–557.

Jones, A. C. Life change and psychological distress as predictors of pregnancy outcome. *Psychosomatic Medicine*, 1978, *40* (5), 402–412.

Kasl, S. V. Issues in patient adherence to health care regimens. *Journal of Human Stress*, 1975, *1* (3), 5–17, 48.

Keller, M. J. Toward a definition of health. *Advances in Nursing Science*, 1981, *4* (1), 43–64.

Kestenbaum, V. *The humanity of the ill.* Knoxville: The University of Tennessee Press, 1982.

Kett, J. F. *The formation of the American medical profession.* New Haven: Yale University Press, 1968.

King, S. H. *Perceptions of illness and medical practice.* New York: Russell Sage Foundation, 1962.

Kiteme, J. Traditional African medicine. In F. X. Grollig, and H. B. Haley (Eds.), *Medical anthropology.* Paris: Mouton Publishers, 1976.

Kleinman, A. Indigenous and traditional systems of healing. In C. Hastings, J. Fadiman, and J. S. Gordon (Eds.), *Health for the whole person.* New York: Bantam Books, Inc., 1981.

Kopelman, L., and Moskop, J. The holistic health movement: A survey and critique. *The Journal of Medicine and Philosophy*, 1981, *6* (2), 209–235.

Kowal, S. J. Emotions as a cause of cancer. *The Psychoanalytic Review*, 1955, *42* (3), 217–227.

Kozier, B., and Erb, G. L. *Fundamentals of nursing: Concepts and procedures.* Menlo Park, California: Addison-Wesley Publishing Company, 1979.

Krantz, D. S., Glass, D. C., Schaeffer, M. A., and Davia, J. E. Behavior patterns and coronary disease: A critical evaluation. In J. T. Cacioppo and R. E. Petty (Eds.), *Perspectives in cardiovascular psychophysiology.* New York: The Guilford Press, 1982.

Kuhn, T. S. *The structure of scientific revolutions* (2nd ed.). Chicago: The University of Chicago Press, 1970.

LaLonde, M. The traditional view of the health field. In P. A. R. Flynn (Ed.), *The healing continuum.* Bowie, Maryland: Robert J. Brady Co., 1980.

Land, D. Food and people: Two systems interacting. In P. Albright and B. P. Albright (Eds.), *Body, mind, and spirit.* Brattleboro, Vermont: The Stephen Greene Press, 1980.

Lange, R. H. Holistic medicine: Is all holistic medicine whole? *New York State Journal of Medicine*, 1980, *80* (6), 996–999.

Lappé, M. Holistic health: A valuable approach to medical care. *The Western Journal of Medicine*, 1979, 131 (6), 475–478.

Lasch, C. *The culture of narcissism*. New York: W.W. Norton & Company, Inc., 1979.

Leavell, H. R. *Preventive medicine for the doctor in his community*. New York: McGraw-Hill Book Company, Inc., 1958.

Leininger, M. The Gadsup of New Guinea and early child-caring behaviors with nursing care implications. In her *Transcultural nursing*. New York: John Wiley & Sons, 1978.

Lemkin, S. R. Holism and socioeconomic reality. *The Western Journal of Medicine*, 1980, *132* (4), 362–363.

Leonard, G. B. Sociological implications of holistic health. *Journal of Holistic Health*, 1978, *3*, 11–15.

LeShan, L. *You can fight for your life*. New York: M. Evans and Company, Inc., 1977.

———. *The mechanic and the gardener*. New York: Holt, Rinehart, and Winston, 1982.

Leventhal, H. Changing attitudes and habits to reduce risk factors in chronic disease. *The American Journal of Cardiology*, 1973, *31* (5), 571–580.

Levine, J. AIDS: Prejudice and progress. *Time*, September 8, 1986, p. 68.

Levine, M. E. Holistic nursing. *Nursing Clinics of North America*, 1971, *6* (2), 253–264.

Levy, S. M. Preface. In her *Biological mediators of behavior and disease: Neoplasia*. New York: Elsevier Science Publishing Company, Inc., 1982.

Lindeboom, G. A. *Descartes and medicine*. Amsterdam: Editions Rodopi N. V., 1978.

Lipowski, Z. J. Holistic-medical foundations of American psychiatry: A bicentennial. *American Journal of Psychiatry*, 1981, *138* (7), 888–895.

Logan, M. H. Humoral medicine in Guatemala and peasant acceptance of modern medicine. In M. H. Logan and E. E. Hunt, Jr. (Eds.), *Health and the human condition: Perspectives on medical anthropology*. North Scituate, Massachusetts: Duxbury Press, 1978.

Luckmann, J., and Sorensen, K. C. (Eds.). *Medical-surgical nursing: A psychophysiologic approach* (2nd ed.). Philadelphia: W. B. Saunders Company, 1980.

McKegney, F. P. Psychosomatic medicine and primary care medicine: Can there be a meeting? *Psychosomatic Medicine*, 1974, *36* (5), 373–376.

McKeown, T. *The role of medicine*. Princeton, New Jersery: Princeton University Press, 1979.

McWhinney, I. R. *An introduction to family medicine*. New York: Oxford University Press, 1981.

Magner, L. N. *A history of the life sciences*. New York: Marcel Dekker, Inc., 1979.

Mandel, I., Franks, P., and Dickinson, J. Improving physician compliance with preventive medicine guidelines. *The Journal of Family Practice*, 1985, *21* (3), 223–224.

Marlatt, G. A. Relapse prevention: A self-control program for the treatment of addictive behaviors. In R. B. Stuart (Ed.), *Adherence, compliance, and generalization in behavioral medicine*. New York: Brunner/Mazel, Publishers, 1982.

Marram, G., Barrett, M. W., and Bevis, E. O. *Primary nursing*. St. Louis: The C. V. Mosby Company, 1979.

Martin, M. J. Tension headache: A psychiatric study. *Headache*, 1966, *6* (2), 47–54.

Masi, A. T. An holistic concept of health and illness: A tricentennial goal for medicine and public health. *Journal of Chronic Diseases*, 1978, *31* (9–10), 563–572.

Maslow, A. H. *Toward a psychology of being* (2nd ed.). New York: D. Van Nostrand Company, 1968.

———. *Motivation and personality* (2nd ed.). New York: Harper & Row, Publishers, 1970.

———. *The farther reaches of human nature*. New York: The Viking Press, 1971.

Matthews, D., and Hingson, R. Improving patient compliance: A guide for physicians. *Medical Clinics of North America*, 1977, *61* (4), 879–889.

Mattson, P. H. *Holistic health in perspective*. Palo Alto, California: Mayfield Publishing Company, 1982.

Mechanic, D. *Medical sociology* (2nd ed.). New York: The Free Press, 1978.

Mendelsohn, R. S. *Confessions of a medical heretic*. New York: Warner Books, Inc., 1979.

Menninger, R. W. Psychiatry 1976: Time for a holistic medicine (Editorial). *Annals of Internal Medicine*, 1976, *84* (5), 603–604.

————. Self-fulfillment: The psychology of personal responsibility. *Journal of Holistic Health*, 1982, *7*, 1–14.

Mikhail, B. The health belief model: A review and critical evaluation of the model, research, and practice. *Advances in Nursing Science*, 1981, *4* (1), 65–80.

Milio, N. A framework for prevention: Changing health-damaging to health-generating life patterns. *American Journal of Public Health*, 1976, *66* (5), 435–439

Miller, J. *The body in question*. New York: Vintage Books, 1982.

Misiak, H., and Sexton, V. S. *Phenomenological, existential, and humanistic psychologies*. New York: Grune & Stratton, 1973.

Moll, J. A. High-level wellness and the nurse. *Topics in Clinical Nursing*, 1982, *3* (4), 61–67.

Monaco, A. J. Coming! Holistic medicine. *Hospital Topics*, 1978, *56* (4), 10–11.

Monmaney, T. Preying on AIDS patients. *Newsweek*, June 1, 1987, pp. 52–54.

Moore, L. G., Van Arsdale, P. W., Glittenberg, J. E., and Aldrich, R. A. *The biocultural basis of health*. St. Louis: The C. V. Mosby Company, 1980.

Morgan, G. W. *The human predicament: Dissolution and wholeness*. Providence, Rhode Island: Brown University Press, 1968.

Moser, R. H. The scientific marketplace and the medical establishment. *The Western Journal of Medicine*, 1980, *132* (2), 160–161.

Multiple Risk Factor Intervention Trial Research Group. Multiple risk factor intervention trial. *Journal of the American Medical Association*, 1982, *248* (12), 1465–1477.

Murdock, G. P. *Theories of illness*. Pittsburgh: University of Pittsburgh Press, 1980.

Narayan, S. M., and Joslin, D. J. Crisis theory and intervention: A critique of the medical model and proposal of a holistic nursing model. *Advances in Nursing Science*, 1980, 2 (4), 27–39.

Nightingale, F. *Notes on nursing*. Chicago: American Health Sciences, 1974.

Noren, J., Frazier, T., Altman, I., and DeLozier, J. Ambulatory medical care. *The New England Journal of Medicine*, 1980, 302 (1), 11–16.

Oleck, L. H., and Yoder, S. D. Holism or hypocrisy? *Perspectives in Psychiatric Care*, 1981, 19 (2), 65–68.

Orvell, B. D. On the etiology of the holistic pseudoschism, *The Western Journal of Medicine*, 1980, 133 (1), 78.

Padrick, K. P. Compliance: Myths and motivators. *Topics in Clinical Nursing*, 1986, 7 (4), 17–22.

Parkerson, G. R., Gehlbach, S. H., Wagner, E. H., James, S. A., Clapp, N. E., and Muhlbaier, L. H. The Duke-UNC health profile: An adult health status instrument for primary care. *Medical Care*, 1981, 19 (8), 806–828.

Parsons, T. Definitions of health and illness in the light of American values and social structure. In E. G. Jaco (Ed.), *Patients, physicians, and illness*. Glencoe, Illinois: The Free Press, 1958.

Passmore, J. *The perfectability of man*. New York: Charles Scribner's Sons, 1970.

Pellegrino, E. D. Being ill and being healed: Some reflections on the grounding of medical morality. In V. Kestenbaum (Ed.), *The humanity of the ill*. Knoxville: The University of Tennessee Press, 1982.

———. Foreword to the English edition: Illness, body, and self. In J. Bergsma and D. C. Thomasma, *Health care: Its psychosocial dimensions*. Pittsburgh: Dusquesne University Press, 1982.

Pelletier, K. R. *Mind as healer, mind as slayer*. New York: Dell Publishing Co., Inc., 1977.

————. *Holistic medicine.* New York: Dell Publishing Co., Inc., 1979a.

————. Holistic medicine: From pathology to prevention. *The Western Journal of Medicine,* 1979b, *131* (6), 481–483.

Penzer, V. Holism: Treating the whole patient. *Journal of the American Dental Association,* 1981, *102* (1), 27–28.

Phillips, D. C. James, Dewey, and the reflex arc. *Journal of the History of Ideas,* 1971, *32* (4), 555–568.

————. *Holistic thought in social science.* Stanford, California: Stanford University Press, 1976.

Pietroni, P. Holistic medicine. *The Journal of the Royal College of General Practitioners,* 1984, *34* (265), 463–464.

Plato. [*Laches and Charmides*] (R. K. Sprague, Trans.). Indianapolis: The Bobbs-Merrill Company, Inc., 1973.

Porkert, M. *The theoretical foundations of Chinese medicine.* Cambridge, Massachusetts: The MIT Press, 1974.

Powell, L. H., Friedman, M., Thoreson, C. E., Gill, J. J., and Ulmer, D. K. Can Type A behavior pattern be altered after myocardial infarction? A second-year report from the recurrent coronary prevention project. *Psychosomatic Medicine,* 1984, *46* (4), 293–313.

Priestman, T. J., Priestman, S. G., and Bradshaw, C. Stress and breast cancer. *The British Journal of Cancer,* 1985, *51* (4), 493–498.

Quintanilla, A. Effect of rural-urban migration on beliefs and attitudes toward disease and medicine in southern Peru. In F. X. Grollig and H. B. Haley (Eds.), *Medical anthropology.* Paris: Mouton Publishers, 1976.

Rather, L. J. *Mind and body in eighteenth century medicine.* London: The Wellcome Historical Medical Library, 1965.

Read, D. A. Holistic health from the inside. *Journal of School Health,* 1983, *53* (6), 382–385.

Reed, J. D. America shapes up. *Time,* November 2, 1981, pp. 94–106.

Rees, W. D., and Lutkins, S. G. Mortality of bereavement. *British Medical Journal,* 1967, *4*, 13–16.

Reich, C. A. *The greening of America.* New York: Random House, 1970.

Reichgott, M. J., and Simons-Morton, B. G. Strategies to improve patient compliance with antihypertensive therapy. *Primary Care*, 1983, *10* (1), 21–27.

Relman, A. S. Holistic medicine (Editorial). *The New England Journal of Medicine*, 1979, *300* (6), 312–313.

Reverby, S. A perspective on the root causes of illness. *American Journal of Public Health*, 1972, *62* (8), 1140–1142.

Rieff, P. *The triumph of the therapeutic.* New York: Harper and Row, Publishers, 1968.

Riscalla, L. M. A holistic concept of the immune system. *Journal of the American Society of Psychosomatic Dentistry and Medicine*, 1983, *30* (3), 97–101.

Rogentine, G. N., van Kammen, D. P., Fox, B. H., Docherty, J. P., Rosenblatt, J. E., Boyd, S. C., and Bunney, W. E. Psychological factors in the prognosis of malignant melanoma: A prospective study. *Psychosomatic Medicine*, 1979, *41* (8), 647–655.

Rogers, C. R. *Carl Rogers on encounter groups.* New York: Harper & Row, 1970.

Rosch, P. J., and Kearney, H. M. Holistic medicine and technology: A modern dialectic. *Social Science & Medicine*, 1985, *21* (12), 1405–1409.

Rosen, G. *Preventive medicine in the United States.* New York: Prodist, 1977.

Rosenblatt, A. D., and Thickstun, J. T. Holistic, field, and humanistic theories (Monograph). *Psychological Issues*, 1978, *11* (2/3), 218–234.

Rosenman, R. H., Brand, R. J., Jenkins, C. D., Friedman, M., Straus, R., and Wurm, M. Coronary heart disease in the Western collaborative group study. *Journal of the American Medical Association*, 1975, *233* (8), 872–877.

Rosenstock, I. M. Why people use health services. *The Milbank Memorial Fund Quarterly*, 1966, Vol. XLIV, No. 3, Part 2, 94–124.

Roszak, T. *The making of a counter culture.* New York: Doubleday & Company, Inc., 1969.

Russell, B. *A history of Western philosophy.* New York: Simon and Schuster, 1945.

Russell, M. A. H., Wilson, C., Taylor, C., and Baker, C. D. Effect of general practitioners' advice against smoking. *British Medical Journal*, 1979, *2*, 231–235.

Ryan, R. S. and Travis, J. W. *The wellness workbook*. Berkeley, California: Ten Speed Press, 1981.

Sabshin, M. On remedicalization and holism in psychiatry. *Psychosomatics*, 1977, *18* (4), 7–8.

Sackett, D. L., and Snow, J. C. The magnitude of compliance and non-compliance. In R. B. Haynes, D. W. Taylor, and D. L. Sackett (Eds.), *Compliance in health care*. Baltimore: The Johns Hopkins University Press, 1979.

Sakalys, J. A. The meanings of health and illness. In P. H. Mitchell (Ed.), *Concepts basic to nursing* (3rd ed.). New York: McGraw-Hill Book Company, 1981.

Salmon, J. W., and Berliner, H. S. Health policy implications of the holistic health movement. *Journal of Health Politics, Policy, and Law*, 1980, *5* (3), 535–553.

Sanders, A. D. Holistic health: What is our response? (Editorial). *Arizona Medicine*, 1979, *36* (3), 203.

Scheffler, I. *The language of education*. Springfield, Illinois: Charles C. Thomas, 1960.

Schloss, G. A., Siroka, R. W., and Siroka, E. K. Some contemporary origins of the personal growth group. In R. W. Siroka, E. K. Siroka, and G. A. Schloss (Eds.), *Sensitivity training and group encounter*. New York: Grosset & Dunlap, 1971.

Schmidt, D. D., Zyzanski, S., Ellner, J., Kumar, M. L., and Arno, J. Stress as a precipitating factor in subjects with recurrent herpes labialis. *The Journal of Family Practice*, 1985, *20* (4), 359–366.

Schrag, C. O. *Experience and being*. Evanston, Illinois: Northwestern University Press, 1969.

Selye, H. A syndrome produced by diverse nocuous agents. *Nature*, 1936, *138* (3479), 32.

———. *The stress of life*. New York: McGraw-Hill Book Company, 1976.

Shafer, K. N., Sawyer, J. R., McCluskey, A. M., and Beck,

E. L. *Medical-surgical nursing* (2nd ed.). St. Louis: The C. V. Mosby Company, 1961.

Shaffer, J. B. P. *Humanistic psychology.* Englewood Cliffs, New Jersey: Prentice-Hall, Inc., 1978.

Shapiro, D., and Goldstein, I. B. Behavioral perspectives on hypertension. *Journal of Consulting and Clinical Psychology,* 1982, *50* (6), 841–858.

Shapiro, J., and Shapiro, D. H. The psychology of responsibility. *The New England Journal of Medicine,* 1979, *301* (4), 211–212.

Shealy, C. N. The psychology of responsibility (Letter). *The New England Journal of Medicine,* 1979, *301* (23), 1294.

Shuval, J. T. The contribution of psychological and social phenomena to an understanding of the aetiology of disease and illness. *Social Science & Medicine,* 1981 *15A* (3), 337–342.

Siegel, B. S., and Siegel, B. H. Holistic medicine. *Connecticut Medicine,* 1981, *45* (7), 441–442.

Siegel, J. M., Johnson, J. H., and Sarason, I. G. Life changes and menstrual discomfort. *Journal of Human Stress,* 1979, *5* (1), 41–46.

Simonton, O. C., Matthews-Simonton, S., and Creighton, J. L. *Getting well again.* New York: Bantam Books, 1980.

Smith, D. The holistic health revolution. *Whole Life Times,* January-February, 1982, p. 21.

Smith, J. A. The idea of health: A philosophical inquiry. *Advances in Nursing Science,* 1981, *3* (3), 43–50.

Smuts, J. C. *Holism and evolution.* New York: Macmillan and Co., 1926.

Snyder, P. *Health and human nature.* Radnor, Pennsylvania: Chilton Book Company, 1980.

Sobel, D. S. Introduction. In D. S. Sobel (Ed.), *Ways of health: Holistic approaches to ancient and contemporary medicine.* New York: Harcourt, Brace, Jovanovich, 1979.

Solomon, P. The x-factor in healing. In P. Albright and B. P. Albright (Eds.), *Body, mind, and spirit.* Brattleboro, Vermont: The Stephen Greene Press, 1980.

Sontag, S. *Illness as metaphor.* New York: Vintage Books, 1979.

Spector, R. E. *Cultural diversity in health and illness.* New York: Appleton-Century-Crofts, 1979.

Spicker, S. F. (Ed.). Introduction. In his *The philosophy of the body: Rejections of Cartesian dualism.* Chicago: Quadrangle Books, 1970.

Stang, J. M., and Stang, O. R. Religion and medicine at the crossroads: (W)holistic health care. *The Ohio State Medical Journal,* 1979, *75* (12), 769–772.

Strauss, B. V. A primer on holistic medical practice. *Connecticut Medicine,* 1978, *42* (9), 557–560.

Suinn, R. M., and Bloom, L. J. Anxiety management training for Pattern A behavior. *Journal of Behavioral Medicine,* 1978, *1* (1), 25–35.

Svihus, R. H. On healing the whole person: A perspective. *The Western Journal of Medicine,* 1979, *131* (6), 478–481.

Taub, S., and Taub, E. A. Health facilitation, a new health-care delivery system that promotes self-responsibility and reduces costs. *Journal of Holistic Health,* 1983, *8,* 1–5.

Thomas, L. On the science and technology of medicine. In J. H. Knowles (Ed.), *Doing better and feeling worse.* New York: W. W. Norton & Company, Inc., 1977.

Tillich, P. The meaning of health. *Perspectives in Biology and Medicine,* 1961, *5* (1), 92–100.

Todd, M. C. Interface: Holistic health and traditional medicine. *The Western Journal of Medicine,* 1979, *131* (6), 464–465.

Travis, J. W. Wellness education and holistic health—How they're related. *Journal of Holistic Health,* 1980a, *3,* 25–32.

———. Wellness education: A new model for health. In P. A. R. Flynn (Ed.), *The healing continuum.* Bowie, Maryland: Robert J. Brady Co., 1980b.

———. Wellness inventory. Reprinted in P. A. R. Flynn, *Holistic health.* Bowie, Maryland: Robert J. Brady Co., 1980c.

Twemlow, S. W., and Chamberlin, C. R. Holistic medicine. *The Journal of the Kansas Medical Society,* 1981, *82* (10), 447–450, 474

U.S. Department of Health, Education, and Welfare/Public Health Service. *Healthy people: The surgeon general's report on health promotion and disease prevention*. DHEW U.S. Government Printing Office (PHS) 79–55071.

Vanderpool, H. Y. The holistic hodgepodge: A critical analysis of holistic medicine and health in America today. *The Journal of Family Practice*, 1984, *19* (6), 773–781.

Vargiu, J., and Remen, N. What is health for? Human priorities in health care. *The Western Journal of Medicine*, 1979, *131* (6), 471–472.

Veith, I. Traditional Chinese medicine: Historical review. In G. B. Risse (Ed.), *Modern China and Traditional Chinese medicine*. Springfield, Illinois: Charles C. Thomas, Publisher, 1973.

Vrooman, J. R. *René Descartes*. New York: G. P. Putnam's Sons, 1970.

Wain, H. *A history of preventive medicine*. Springfield, Illinois: Charles C. Thomas, Publisher, 1970.

Wallis, R., and Morley, P. (Eds.). Introduction. In their *Marginal medicine*. New York: The Free Press, 1976.

Warner, K. E. Selling health promotion to corporate America. *Health Education Quarterly*, 1987, *14* (1), 39–55.

Watson, W. G. A holistic approach to malpractice—Informed consent (Editorial). *American Journal of Orthodontics*, 1979, *76* (4), 458–461.

Weil, A. *Health and healing*. Boston: Houghton Mifflin Company, 1983.

Wershow, H. J., and Reinhart, G. Life change and hospitalization: A heretical view. *Journal of Psychosomatic Research*, 1974, *18* (6), 393–401.

White, G. E. Strategies in self-image and holistic health. *The Journal of Pedodontics*, 1980, *5* (1), 72–76.

Whorton, J. C. *Crusaders for fitness*. Princeton, New Jersey: Princeton University Press, 1982.

Will, G. F. Dr. Koop's R_x for violence. *Boston Sunday Globe*, November 14, 1982, p. A27.

Williams, N. A., and Deffenbacher, J. L. Life stress and chronic yeast infections. *Journal of Human Stress*, 1983, *9* (1), 26–31.

Wittkower, E. D. A retrospective look at psychosomatic medicine. *Canadian Psychiatric Association Journal*, 1972, *17* (1), 1–2.

Wood, C. S. *Human sickness and health*. Palo Alto, California: Mayfield Publishing Company, 1979.

Wooley, A. S. Defining the product of baccalaureate education. *Nursing and Health Care*, 1986, *7* (4), 199–201.

World Health Organization. *Constitution: World Health Organization*. Geneva: 1947.

Yahn, G. The impact of holistic medicine, medical groups, and health concepts. *Journal of the American Medical Association*, 1979, *242* (20), 2202–2205.

Zaner, R. M. *The context of self: A phenomenological inquiry using medicine as a clue*. Athens, Ohio: Ohio University Press, 1981.

Zbilut, J. P. Holistic nursing: The transcendental factor. *Nursing Forum*, 1980, *19* (1), 45–49.

Zorn, F. *Mars*. New York: Alfred A. Knopf, 1982.

Zucker, A. Holism and reductionism: A view from genetics. *The Journal of Medicine and Philosophy*, 1981, *6* (2), 145–163.

Index